The
Healing
Journey
A Workbook For
Self-Discovery

MARK PEARSON began teaching primary school in NSW, then founded a remedial reading clinic. For five years he held a senior staff position at the Living Water Centre, Blue Mountains, NSW, as lecturer in emotional release counselling for children, transpersonal breathwork, dreamwork and other ERC methods.

He has a special interest in the body, mind, emotion connection in the healing process. He enjoys supporting the expression of emerging wholeness in creative new ways that are in tune with an individual's deeper purpose.

He works as a psychotherapy and counselling trainer, directing courses and personal development programmes at 'The Portiuncula' Centre, in Toowoomba, 'The New Heart Centre', Rockhampton, for the Australian Council for Educational Research (ACER), in Melbourne, and through Turnaround Personal Development Programmes in Brisbane.

He is the co-author (with Patricia Nolan) of *Emotional First-Aid For Children* (1991) and *Emotional Release For Children* (1995) and author of the first Australian book on Breathwork: *From Healing To Awakening* (1991). He has a new book in preparation on self-esteem and self-awareness for children and adolescents.

Mark is a founding member of the NSW and Qld Emotional Release Counsellors Associations.

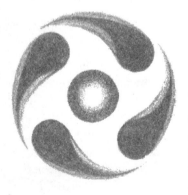

This mandala shows four energy circles revolving around a centre. All parts of life are in movement and flow:

- love, relationships and sexuality
- outer work, career, mission
- play, rest, entertainment
- spiritual practice, the healing journey, self-discovery.

When all these parts are alive and active they create the energy of the centre—the self. Life is flow and movement.

Designed by Mark Pearson and illustrated by Lynette Fox.

The Healing Journey

A Workbook For Self-Discovery

Mark Pearson

Lothian
B O O K S

The self-discovery questions and exercises in this book are in no way intended as a substitute for professional support in the area of personal growth, counselling or therapy.

Working with these exercises may in fact activate your wish to further your healing journey and seek experienced support. Some questions may upset you; they may challenge your self-image and reactivate old memories which are holding you back. They may reveal a new level of feelings and help you remember who you really are.

Thomas C. Lothian Pty Ltd
11 Munro Street, Port Melbourne, Victoria 3207
Copyright © Mark Pearson 1997

First published 1997

National Library of Australia
Cataloguing-in-Publication data:
    Pearson, Mark.
    The healing journey.
    Includes index
    ISBN 0 85091 853 7.
    1. Adjustment (Psychology). 2. Emotions.
    3. Suffering.
    I. Title
152.4

Cover design and illustration by Trudi Canavan
Photography by Tess Pearson
Typeset in Australia by Melbourne Media Services
Printed in Australia by McPherson's Printing Group

Contents

Acknowledgments

Ahrara Carisbrooke — for the years of teaching and encouragement with personal healing and the journey.

Karen Daniel — for partnership in developing inner work methods.

Rosemary Pearson — for her love and keen eye that again saved me grammatical and spelling embarrassments; and for offering valuable suggestions and challenging questions on the first draft.

Patricia Nolan — for the creative mind, being a sounding-board, a source of many new ideas and an unrelenting enthusiast for the value of inner work.

Pat Quinn, Mary Madden and Helen Wilson — the Portiuncula team — for providing the place, the times, the challenges and feedback that refined the ways inner work can be taught.

Trainees and Clients — for the privilege of sharing in their journeys and giving feedback on developing methods.

The Emotional Release Counsellors professional associations — for bringing order to the way the inner work is conducted and taught.

The personal growth pioneers and consciousness researchers such as Stan and Christina Grof, C. G. Jung, Wilhelm Reich, Fritz Perls, Arthur Janov and particularly Eva Pierrakos, as well as many others, from whose work so much healing and so many methods and inspiration have been drawn. Especially to Stan Grof who helps us experience the connection between our personal inner work and the cosmic possibilities.

Tess Pearson for photography.

How can we remember who we really are?

How can we remember that under the load of our personal struggles,
under our childhood hurts and initial shock in meeting this world,
lies the memory of who we are, where we came from,
why we are here now?

Under our education, and all the roles of personality,
under the imprints that shape our character,
under the moulding, the masks and the manners,
lies our essence.

Under the amusements and distractions, under the endless thoughts
and aches and pain, beneath our moods and our postures,
lies the pure vibration of life.

Under confusion, under armour, ideals and divisions,
beyond persona, ego, and shadow,
lies our wholeness.

Under the struggle to make a living, under the search for a mate,
under the duties and chores and routines,
lies our special contribution.

Under the daydreams and fantasies,
under the wishing, the waiting for magic,
lies our work for consciousness.
Deep down, under the label of our profession,
under 'parent', under 'partner',
lies our real purpose.

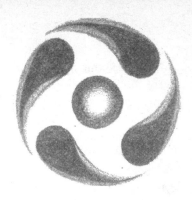

Preface

One of the most fulfilling aspects of my life at the moment is working with groups, encouraging inner growth and offering training in some practical personal development methods. From time to time, I recognise a sense of 'mission' in sharing these inner growth methods, and this book exists to satisfy that part of me.

I have been well supported by many colleagues and friends. I live in a community in which vulnerability can emerge, and where the awakening of my shadow side does not bring condemnation. An understanding and supportive environment will always point you back to the source — to the healer within yourself. This is precious and rare. This support makes the journey possible.

Patricia Nolan and I were delighted that our first book *Emotional First-Aid for Children* (1991) sold out within its first year of publication. What we thought was a very specialised and challenging text was widely and enthusiastically received, not only by counsellors who work with children, but by teachers, tertiary lecturers, parents and counsellors who work with adults. All were eager for more support, more knowledge, more methods. We were pleased that it has been reprinted and that the sequel *Emotional Release For Children* (1995) has been published and is also well received.

The approaches we explore in this book range from quiet pondering and meditation to dramatic emotional release and new awareness. Underlying the methods (and driving me on) is the growing knowledge of a new alive way of being in the world that is both very practical and subtly spiritual.

In times gone by our practical side and our spiritual nature were thought of as separate. The present times demand a new approach: creative, positive action in the world, informed by a spiritual energy and knowledge. This conscious action needs to come from much more than just our egoic selves.

The great ways that directed human inner growth through the ages sometimes seem less accessible to modern people. Most of us have our personal problems so much to the fore that the ways of hope, faith, love and meditation seem to have little impact.

This book is based on the methods of self-discovery and emotional first-aid for adults belonging to what we call Emotional Release Counselling. ERC includes a wide range of approaches that address our personal problems and bring harmony between the conscious and the unconscious — between the inner world of the psyche and outer life. This eventually brings more harmony in the so-called 'real' social, political external world. And, being informed by a spiritual approach, ERC also begins to bring forth deep contact with essence or soul. This often feels like a flow of subtle energies in the body. It is our first real experience of what has been called the divine. The great internal distance we feel from the divine flow, or meaninglessness, has often been cited as the main 'illness' of the twentieth century.

There are, of course, more stages of inner work, other spiritual disciplines, that go beyond the scope of Emotional Release Counselling. These stages become more accessible, more understandable, more desirable and more possible after the backlog of our personal miseries and misunderstandings has been cleared.

I see the inner work methods of Emotional Release Counselling as embodying the practical side of many of the world's great teachings on personal and spiritual growth. The ulations presented in this book are a harvest pro- the labours of many people trying to understand , to reduce their inner suffering and share what them.

us are afraid of knowing and showing who we creatures made in the likeness of the divine. Our e link between our human and divine origins —

has been covered over. It has been covered by fear, grief, anger and hatred. We have grown up to believe ourselves to be fearful, grieving, angry or hateful people.

Under those external layers we are really compassionate, aware, tender and able to love. When we return to our deep ability to feel we reconnect with the energy of our whole self and the divine — which has always permeated us and surrounded us. Encouraging the movement towards this essential level is the aim of the ideas and exercises in this book.

Through travels to workshops and training groups around Australia and in New Zealand, I have seen that there is a strong emerging call. Those who have really begun the journey of uncovering their truth are called to begin to show it in daily life; to show who they really are. The call is built into each of us. Many now answer the call through journeying, training and then going into practice as counsellors and therapists. Others find ways that are in tune with their particular gifts. All who gain from this inner work eventually begin to radiate a positive, hopeful, energy, whether they intend it or not. This is a very precious and scarce commodity!

My hope is that in *The Healing Journey* you may discover some keys that begin to unlock the prisons of suffering that so many of us find ourselves in. The keys have been cast and recast down through the ages and these new ones are designed to fit the present locks we find within. There are ideas and questions to put us in touch with the strong heroic person inside who can use the keys. For many of us — for the planet perhaps — it is urgent that the keys be used. May they never get rusty!

Mark Pearson
Brisbane

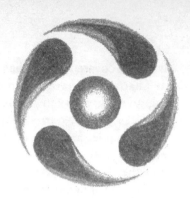

Introduction

Seeking help to understand your inner world and seeking counselling to heal it are signs of health. In the past the need for support in the areas of mental and emotional health was seen as a sign of ill-health. It is obvious now that disregarding your inner world, putting on a brave face, and denying your vulnerability can lead to disastrous consequences.

At the same time you do not have to be a vulnerable victim in life. You can be fully responsible for yourself because you are capable of healing and growth, and opening to the fullness of your potential. In fact it is your responsibility to grow. The planet urgently needs more people to grow up, to heal and then contribute in a mature way.

In my personal growth work over many years I have seen so many people emerge from a state of deep emotional brokenness to being able and ready to support others. They become able to contribute their unique skills, outlook and creativity, and add much to the welfare of others.

This book is about starting that journey of healing. Each of us is called at some time to face the past, to release it, and then find the methods and support to turn around and face the future and recognise what we have to offer. This book introduces some helpful and probing questions and methods. You can use the questions and journal exercises alone or with your partner or, better still, form a small group of seekers to share discoveries with.

The work in this book is based on Emotional Release Counselling. ERC is a formulation of effective counselling and personal growth methods that has been developed in Australia from clinical work and transpersonal and sacred psychology. It includes a range of traditional and process-oriented methods that explore unconscious self-images, beliefs and habitual ways of being. The underlying principle of ERC is to bring emotional healing and clarity for adults, adolescents and children.

The main modalities of ERC are emotional release processing, transpersonal breathwork, sandplay, symbol work, dreamwork, bioenergetics, journal writing, mandala symbolism and meditation.

Everyone carries emotional imprints from the past and although these are not seen, they are operative and can have a negative effect on the way you live your life. You are defended against unpleasant memories and feelings from the past, yet they remain inside you causing unfulfilling, and even destructive, emotional and lifestyle patterns. These old feelings, along with present reactions, can be fully felt, mobilised, worked with, expressed and released safely. This results in a new inner connection to self and a clearer, more direct, relationship to those around you.

The inner-life skills component of ERC brings deep and lasting feelings of self-esteem and self-awareness. There are seven broad areas of the inner-life skills:

- self-knowledge
- understanding the unconscious
- self-expression and communication
- managed emotional and physical release
- relating to others
- supporting others, and
- understanding our own motivation and direction in life.

This book is designed to bring you insight that supports emotional and psychological healing. It is intended as a bridge between the sometimes awesome depths of transpersonal therapies and the first self-awareness that flows from quiet pondering, journal writing, exploring dreams and reading and reflecting on maps for the healing journey.

It is appropriate to caution you too because this book is designed to provoke responses, upset self-images and support the long-term process of emotional release and healing. If you take responsibility for your reactions to the questions — that is, find a new ability to respond — the journey will have begun. Hopefully *The Healing Journey* will stir up your hunger for a better way of being in the world; and inspire hope that this is really possible.

Those of us who find ourselves connected with a group of fellow searchers are in the best position to allow deep healing work, transformation, and eventually inner harmony. The creation of new community for the purpose of healing may be your new aim. Receiving the support of others will help you realise that the most important place you can make real changes is within. The starting place for all the changes the world needs is you.

Every person is valuable and needed; each person has something to give. You are not really an isolated ego, but an alive, individual particle of the whole. The world needs hope. Hope comes from seeing models of positive transformation, alive energy and peace. These things only exist in individuals.

All traditions suggest that for your inner work to bear fruit and ripen, you must dedicate it to the good of all. At a certain stage of your healing you become able to see beyond personal needs. You emerge from your cocoon of personal issues, personal pain and begin to see and respond to the implications beyond yourself. Personal healing benefits your partner, friends, children and family, your community and possibly the planet.

The more you heal and come to wholeness, the more you can give. You can give through actions in the world, and through radiating a positive inner being. This positive and creative inner being is a true reflection of the divine and of the way life was meant to be. It awakens the same spark in others.

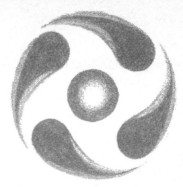

1

Maps for the Journey
AN OVERVIEW OF METHODS AND APPROACHES

We are concerned, are we not, with the exploration
of our inward nature which is very complex.
This investigation is really self-education —
not to change what is, but to understand what is.
What is, is far more important than what should be.
The understanding of what we actually are
is far more essential than to transcend what we are.

J. Krishnamurti from *Letters To The Schools* Vol. 2 (1985)

Emotional release counselling and self-discovery as a journey

Soon after birth we begin to drift apart from a deep connection with a special, divine energy. Many people who pursue a healing journey report remembering this connection and knowing that very deep in their unconscious the link has not been broken, just covered over by the shock of birth and the disappointments of early life. When you are born your essence, your potential, is usually intact and ready to develop.

To defend yourself from physical and emotional pain, and to lessen the shock of coming out into a world that falls so far short of expectations, you repress your feelings. This unconscious process of repression is compounded as you contract your muscles, reduce your breath and dull your sensations.

1

Repression helps you survive, but it begins the disconnection with your inner life.

Growing up is often a process of learning inner and outer defences against feeling hurt, separate, unseen and unmet. The inner defences are hormonal, neurological, muscular and respiratory. Your reactions of anger, rage and hate are locked away in what Jung has called the shadow, away from consciousness. But along with these strong reactions you lock up large amounts of energy and, from then on, you also have to use large amounts of energy to keep things locked up. Frequently our unmet tenderness is stored away too.

In learning what is not acceptable you also learn what way of being is considered ideal. Many of us develop an idealised self-image. This is an image of what we think our parents would like us to be — the way that wins love and approval. You may fight this idealised self-image by running away, dyeing your hair blue or dropping out. Rebelling against your parents for imposing this ideal may be your main motivation. As an adolescent and adult you may unconsciously embroider this ideal self, enlarge it and strive to uphold it. It is possible to spend a lifetime struggling to attain this image and suffering from your perceived shortcomings, or sabotaging your life by fighting against it.

Wilhelm Reich, an early explorer of contemporary body and emotion-oriented therapies, uses the term 'armouring' for the chronic muscular tension that we all develop. In some cases this armouring begins after only a few weeks out in the world. It constricts the flow of your emotions, inhibits unacceptable movements, controls excitement, and eventually drains your personal energy. If one feeling is held down then to some degree everything in us is held down. Since it is only through a deep flowing of personal energy that we connect with and experience the sacred, we often are disconnected from much of our spiritual potential.

Each time your emotional and physical needs are not met a part of you closes in. An inner child forms, made up of incomplete feelings, of feelings that were too painful to feel, of longings too strong to bear and traumas too upsetting to stay in consciousness. The positive, joy-filled aspects of life tend to be welcomed in, but there is a separation within, a hurt inner child, a separate persona. This child part is fixated on what it did not get and keeps looking for the recognition, approval and comfort that it did not receive. It seeks compensations or indirect ways of obtaining pleasure from the world.

Your ego is the sum of your inner child, your idealised self-image, your armouring, your defences and need for compensations. By adulthood you are probably several steps removed from your essence and living according to the dictates of the outer world. Habits become set in an attempt to extract what you need within yourself from the outside world. Since you lose contact with an authentic base inside yourself, a struggle to strengthen the ego takes over. You try to grow up as quickly as possible into what looks 'adult' from the outside.

Out of this false, moulded ego you set up your life — careers, relationships, struggles. But your essence is not nourished and it ceases to grow, to be known or listened to. To the degree you are distant from your essence this outer endeavour must be unfulfilling. We all eventually become accustomed to quietening the inner longing and not stopping to listen to our inner life.

However, at some point in most people's lives this tight grip on the repressed inner life seems to weaken. The locks on the gates that have held back undesired memories tend to break. If this unconscious material from the past bursts forth too quickly the person may suffer a 'nervous breakdown' because they can no longer sustain the strain of maintaining an unhealthy ego structure. For many this weakening of emotional repression begins in the mid-thirties, sometimes earlier, often later. The so-called mid-life crisis is very much this conflict between the old pains, the unfulfilling life we have set up, and the absence of real meaning which alone comes from being connected to the flow of energy through the body.

Sometimes a spiritual awakening, a moment of special grace, will stimulate you to begin a serious search for what is wrong with your life. For some the inner revolt grows quietly and steadily supported by a search through the literature on growth and purpose.

As the need for inner growth is aroused people begin to drop some of the defences that they spent so long cultivating. They begin to allow some vulnerability and perhaps look around for books, friends or professionals in the personal growth areas. Although there may be a resonance with the traditional ways or religions those sources may not be particularly helpful at the moment. Some New Age approaches focus very much on the 'light', but the need at this stage is to thoroughly know the dark as well. Traditional psychology and psychiatry may help strengthen the ego to get back to what the world considers a stable way of living. But most of us want more than that.

If a strong need to discover and release your real self emerges here and if that need meets the right support, you begin what some call the Introvert Stage of your healing journey. This involves really dealing with yourself. It is the right time to find approaches that meet you exactly where you are and support you to release the burden of the past and rediscover the abundance of the present. ERC, breathwork and quiet meditation combine with a sense of being ready, and gradually you remember, feel and express all your old pains, rage and hate. The healing journey begins with loosening your armouring, reclaiming energy from the shadow, and feeling what you could not feel as a child. This diminishes the power of the inner child to spoil your adult life. You become more ready and able to make the outer changes you know you need.

The healing and transformation taking place inside causes the ego to crumble and your old coping mechanisms are far less effective. From the outside, to those who do not understand, it seems as if you are going backwards. You are more vulnerable to the pressures you have set up in your life.

These times of feeling more real become very precious. The energy of reality, of true and strong emotions, of lifeforce in your body, begins to attract you more than the old pretence. It can be a lonely time as those around you may be forced to change too or retreat a little from you. It can be a time of challenge to your careers, relationships and families. Most of the world is established by and caters for egos that want predictable outcomes, and you are beginning to let our life be motivated by something deep inside, something that might love change, growth and new life.

When your personal healing work extends into the journey that gives meaning to your whole life you know that you are in the process that Jung called individuation — becoming an individual, truly who you were meant to become. At this time you have more contact with your essence; your 'being' grows and you may recognise that too much of your life has been 'doing'. Now you are ready to explore a more simple life; one that really nourishes you, one that welcomes 'being'.

Many emotional release processes take you through a profound experience in which your ego crumbles but at the same time you find a new structuring principle that comes from the freed up energy and from your essence. As this happens the ego begins to take its rightful place as a servant, rather than having us believe it is the master.

The feeling of being at home in your body, present and vividly alive, increases in duration and frequency and you find a new creativity. This extra energy, this surplus, means that you are ready for the Extrovert Stage, which is a time to explore giving back to others and to the world. At this time you can continue your inner healing work, perhaps in a more subtle way, and begin to find ways of helping others. We find we have love to spare! There is usually a call from within to help in some way, either directly with support for other people's inner growth, or in some other way that matches our particular gifts.

Of course, there are people who are active extroverts in their career. When they come to this stage in their healing journey they will begin to take much more time for themselves. They will be able to offer support without having to; they can allow it to happen instead of doing by compulsion.

Even if your particular way of giving seems small, the fact that you are able to give now, and are no longer totally consumed by your neediness, is a huge and socially important step.

Underlying this stage is the challenge of moving into a fulfilling lifestyle. The excitement grows as you taste the possibility of knowing and getting what you really need. No one deeply needs a million dollars. You don't really need Mr or Ms Perfect to appear to make you whole. You may be open to abundance and new relationships, but your new skill is also in finding fulfilment within and with the simple things around.

As you approach the end of the healing journey your ability to support others grows. You become interested in the effort — but not the struggle — to give something back. Your path and the ways of growth that attract you come closer to resembling the traditional ways. Life becomes simpler. You enjoy loving rather than seeking love.

From this stage that is characterised by growing happiness and well-being, as well as a new willingness to face challenges, you may search out new ways and new levels within that are beyond the modalities of ERC. They may be methods, like meditation, that you tried in the past, but which failed to address your personal needs. Since you are mature at last, these traditional ways can now be more effective.

Some requirements for happiness

Many of us have learned to accept unhappiness, or limited happiness, as our basic condition. We began to learn this in childhood, and it has become so pervasive that we hardly notice it. This limited belief system holds us back from searching further for a way out and from achieving our full potential. I am not implying that life should only be happy, but unfortunately so many of us accept a continuous background state of worry, depression, struggle and unfulfilment.

The healing journey leads you through some emotional pain in order to create inner space for experiences of happiness, moments of well-being, states of balance and pleasure. You will then have something to measure the rest of your life against. To experience deeply a happy time can be disturbing. This disturbance can help your journey if you understand it. Feeling unsettled or upset arises from the perception of contrasts and it is part of the price you may have to pay for healing and self-discovery.

You have a lot of unlearning to do! Your hurt inner child part has often been told to accept what it has, and be grateful. Gradually you will learn that you have a right to be happy and to experience times of peace, calm, pleasure and spiritual connection. In recognising this right you are mobilised to

The Healing Journey

Connection with the divine

↓

Birth shock

↓

Childhood — develop ego —learn to bury feelings —
defend against lacks, hurts or trauma
Learn limiting beliefs about self

Expect love to come to us from the outside

↓

Live according to outer world requirements:

Adolescence — Search for role models and wisdom figures

↓

Adult — conflict and stress between inner and outer
world, sabotage by hurt inner child

↙ ↓ ↘ →

Growing dissatisfaction, spiritual awakening, change, loss or crisis

↓

Introvert stage:

Begin search for healing and meaning — focus on self-healing

↓

Release of past, becoming undefended, ego shift

↓

Bring outer life into harmony with inner life

↓

Taste of our real potential

Learn self love

↓

Extrovert stage:

Able and ready to give love

Fulfilment, wholeness, excitement — spiritual practice

↓

Live according to spiritual direction

↓

Reconnect with the divine

search for ways of living that lead you to achieve the requirements for happiness.

These are some of the inner requirements for times of
happiness:

1 Free-flowing personal energy. You need to have your body
  alive, your feelings awake and your attention focussed. You
  must learn to become responsible for your personal energy.

2 Free expression of emotion. This is threefold:

   • having the knowledge and experience to transform nega-
     tive emotions into positive ones;

   • overcoming the fear of feeling and expressing feelings;

   • recognising the difference between feelings that are true,
     present, adult emotions and those that come from the
     past, from the child. The adult feelings need to be shared
     and expressed; the child ones need to be processed
     through ERC methods. Understanding this distinction is
     vital, especially in our personal relationships.

3 Speaking your truth — not hiding what you think or
  believe. This makes you whole inside even though it may
  upset others or disturb their lives. Again clarity is needed
  around what is present and what is from the past.

4 Living your truth. This includes becoming sincere with
  yourself; being real in relationships; acceptance of change,
  the birth of the new, remembering that whatever is alive is
  changing; 'paying our way in the world'; finding satisfaction from outer work and what it contributes; finding a
  career that is in tune with your real self.

5 Discovering or remembering your deepest purpose and
  moving toward living it! For most this is an ongoing
  search.

6 Taking responsibility for your energy. You begin to honour
  and recognise your own energy as a source or basis for happiness and spirituality. This includes the gradual giving up
  of believing something 'out there' is going to make things
  right within you.

7 Beginning inner healing work. You need to find a new routine in daily life that gives time for your personal energy
  to be free and for it to connect with another energy both
  beyond and within us — the divine. At first this may mean
  an ERC processing time, but later it may become a more

subtle meditation time, a simple tuning in with inner focus. For most of us this time for ourselves has been, and remains, last on the list in a busy life.

Maybe all this sounds like a giant task? It must be clear that the happiness we are talking about is not something cheap or easy. It is a deep foundation within, a gradually evolving platform that supports the activities, the endeavours, the aims of your life. This inner work is to heal wounding and release personal energy as a preparation for forming a lasting basis for a new level of happiness and composure.

Three levels of psychology

The effectiveness of contemporary healing methods now in use owes much to the coming together of three levels of psychology. ERC blends and draws from these three levels.

We categorise the three levels as:

1 Clinical and academic psychology
2 Transpersonal psychology
3 Sacred psychology.

These terms do not relate exclusively to any one modality or belong to any one theorist, but cover a range of theories, methods and knowledge both modern and ancient. ERC draws much from each level. The journey of any individual could be plotted on a graph representing the relationships of these levels and showing the individual's growth from the first level to the third level. In discussing these levels we will have to use many generalisations, and there will always be some exceptions.

The three psychologies relate to different levels of experience and different levels of consciousness. In essence, the three levels do not contradict each other, but have a progressively wider view of the psyche and of the flow and maintenance of human energy. Each level also has its own 'laws'. The laws that are rational and provable are different for each level.

Each successive level embodies more subtle ways of knowing, more direct and objective ways of self-knowledge.

Whereas much of the knowledge of the first level is based on intellectual processes, the second level knowledge comes from the emotions and body awareness as well as the intellect. Those people who begin to know the third level report, as do the sacred books of all the great traditions, a way of knowing, a way of consciousness that includes first and second level knowledge and other higher functions of the human psyche not normally accessed. These higher functions can connect people with degrees of consciousness that seem beyond the limits of human functioning. Jung, for example, explored and wrote about the possible connection to the collective unconscious. His explorations took him from Level 1, where he began along with colleagues such as Freud, through Level 2, towards Level 3.

Level 1 collects its data from what can be perceived by the senses in an ordinary state of consciousness. This 'ordinary' state of consciousness would seem extremely limited from the viewpoint of Levels 2 and 3. Knowledge on Level 2 is gathered by what is available to the five senses as well as what is perceived by other more subtle senses in a non-ordinary state of consciousness. Although these higher levels of consciousness might be dismissed by Level 1, they are in fact the result of a more holistic search and an acquired, refined energy that fuels expanded consciousness.

The knowledge and wisdom of Level 3 is probably impossible to assess from the lower levels. It comes from a higher level which incorporates all that is known in the two lower levels as well as what humans are capable of in their full development — in their completed evolution. When truly embodied, this third level is taught by those who have achieved harmonious functioning of body, mind and feelings, and who have opened to the higher parts of the psyche. From the lower levels, the activation of energy bodies and higher functions of the brain may seem like supernatural abilities, or even be interpreted by some rigid thinkers as symptoms of pathology!

Someone who has been fully engaged in their inner quest and moved through personal emotional healing, and persevered, may find the right support to move from Level 1 to 2, then on towards Level 3.

Level one

Academic or clinical psychology spans the development of the psyche from birth to death. Relevant data is collected from what can be perceived by the senses in an ordinary state of consciousness. This level honours clear thought and reason. Its laws of reason are based only on its own level. Level 1 thinking doubts and frequently scoffs at the idea of higher states or non-ordinary states of consciousness. It tends to ignore the vastness and widespread impact of repressed memories and feelings in the unconscious. Level 1 practitioners are often afraid of the stronger human emotions.

Most importantly, the first level thinkers, writers and practitioners often regard the average repressed person as 'normal'. The data of this level is based on the study of repressed people. It studies people as they are, in their unevolved, sometimes unbalanced states.

There is much new evidence, based on the discoveries of transpersonal psychology, that some symptoms that were previously given psychiatric labels — assessed by Level 1 practitioners — are actually a breakthrough of transpersonal, or Level 2, experiences. The support and treatment methods developed by Level 2 practitioners for people going through these experiences enables them to be integrated and become evolutionary experiences for the psyche. This support is not available from Level 1.

It is normal for those working with Level 1 healing modalities to be engaged in analysis for many years. Level 1 practitioners usually regard transformation and healing as long slow processes. Many of us begin our healing journey with Level 1 modalities and frameworks and then acquire a hunger for the more holistic and effective Level 2 and 3 approaches.

Emotional Release Counselling has been developed to support that hunger by practitioners and seekers who are also moving towards the transpersonal and sacred dimensions of life. They have not been satisfied with Level 1 aims or methods.

Functioning in a way that seems normal in society is an aim of Level 1 inner work. To achieve this it may support inner defences and bolster ego-strength. Level 1 may not recognise anything higher than the ego. For a long time Level 1 psychology only recognised the so-called modern approaches — twentieth century, but not too recent!

Jung and Reich, who developed their exploration and knowledge beyond Level 1 to Level 2, and even began to approach Level 3, were largely ignored by Level 1 psychologists until recently. Only their work that conformed to Level 1 ideology was widely accepted and studied.

ERC has been developed to take you further than Level 1 methods. This book is designed to awaken or support your hunger for more effective and holistic ways for personal and spiritual growth.

Level two

Transpersonal psychology has many definitions. It integrates modern consciousness research with ancient methods and outlooks. From the perspective of higher or non-ordinary states of consciousness it can recognise the links between spiritual and psychological systems and teachings from the present and past. It tends to integrate rather than separate. It accepts experiences that come from a higher level or higher parts of the psyche that may be considered pathological to Level 1 and the modern medical profession.

Researchers who work at this level tend to be seekers themselves and so have personally experienced the healing journey. They are comfortable with awakening and utilising the full energy of the emotions. Because of this the fear of the strong emotions, often found amongst Level 1 practitioners, is almost entirely reduced. Without this fear more emotion can be released and healed. Basic trust in the goodness and order of the psyche enables braver and bolder research.

Without this fear of feelings those working at Level 2 can open to the full range of human experience which includes transpersonal or spiritual energies and experiences — what to many are considered non-ordinary states. The importance of these deeper energies in the healing process is recognised. First the body, feelings and mind have to be engaged in the healing process, then another energy is awakened that can reorder and heal. This other energy has many names in many cultures. It has been connected to nature, to God. It has nothing to do with belief or religion, although religions have been built around this energy. Because of the opening to this superior healing force transformation and healing frequently occurs during Level 2 inner work. Moments of transformation are often quick processes, and can often result in major personality changes. These changes are seen as good and natural, although they may disturb the outer life of the person.

Some of the main pioneers of Level 2 are Dr Stanislav Grof and Christina Grof. Dr Grof began his psychiatric work using first level methods then he researched non-ordinary states of consciousness induced by LSD. Later he and his wife Christina developed Holotropic Breathwork, a natural method of opening to transpersonal dimensions. It seems their current direction is leading more towards discoveries and understanding of Level 3.

Dr Arthur Janov extended our understanding of Level 1 in his work with primal therapy. His major contribution to the understanding of the effects of birth and infancy have helped many, including Dr Frederick Leboyer. Janov, however, denied the transpersonal or spiritual levels, which some who have used his methods now wish to open.

Dr C. G. Jung worked as a colleague of Freud. Based on his clinical observations and his own fearless self-enquiry, he tried to bridge Level 1 and Level 3 and charted the levels of consciousness in Level 2.

Dr Wilhelm Reich's work has had, and continues to have, a strong influence. It is carried forward by many psychologists and personal growth explorers. He began with Level 1 and extended its boundaries until he recognised Level 2. He comprehended aspects of Level 3, but this part of his work was not taken seriously by most contemporaries.

Level three

Sacred psychology is something that is ever-present, but at the same time it remains in the background. There have been many attempts to encompass what it is, to understand the way it works and find methods to move towards it. It is so vast that any one aspect of Level 3 can become the life-time work of a seeker or psychological researcher. Obviously it can only be known in fragments because comprehension of its totality would imply a level of consciousness broader and finer than that in which we normally live.

Methods of attaining the sacred level of consciousness, the interpretations and outer forms for passing it on, have changed with the times, but the core knowledge remains the same. It is often available through myths and teaching stories. Its influence is more obvious in eastern cultures and native indigenous cultures.

Level 3 comes from a higher, evolved consciousness so it includes knowledge of possible human evolution and what we could be when whole and complete. The forms of sacred psychology have been restated and reformulated for this century by G. I. Gurdjieff. Down through the ages mystics and also scientists who have been able to transcend the limits of their ego have described aspects of sacred psychology.

Many consciousness explorers are working with the links between the levels and recognising that personal healing is so much more effective when conducted in the light of spiritual or transpersonal growth. This form of spirituality is not encumbered with the dogmas, beliefs, superstitions and rules that have surrounded, and made heavy, human efforts to capture the spiritual in organised religion, consciousness movements or cults. The spirituality of Level 2 and Level 3 is pure and comes from personal experience that is natural and intrinsic.

There is a tendency for new personal growth movements to try to leap between the three levels and mix them up, often without any consistency or true guidance. They mix belief with knowledge, materialism with spirituality and ego with essence. In many cases the concepts from higher levels are being utilised by the ego with all its limitations.

The world needs more of the influence of Level 3 to help balance the apparent decline in the level of 'being' in society. This decline is evident in the effect humans are having on nature and on the planet. There is much evidence around us now that understanding and interest in Level 3 is expanding.

There is a growing power in the numbers of people beginning their search, their healing, their self-discovery, and

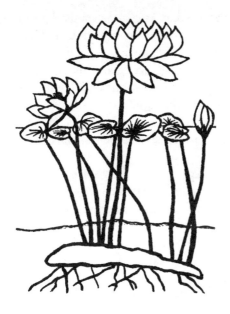

The lotus plant is often used as a symbol for the spiritual journey.

moving towards the higher levels. It is our hope that this force becomes more and more effective in the world.

The basic principles of emotional release counselling

The image of a lotus plant in full flower has been used in some eastern cultures as a symbol for the spiritual journey. It can symbolise the connection between matter — the mud at the bottom of the pond — and spirit — the air and the sun above. I would like to use this symbol here as a basis for introducing some of the concepts and principles of the healing journey with ERC.

The lotus is similar to a waterlily which you may be more familiar with in Australia, except that it rises up above the water held firmly on a strong stem. Its roots are in the mud but the stem carries the bud which reaches up to the warmth and light, and finally opens into a many-petalled flower. The broad green leaves float on the water gathering energy. The three mediums in which the plant lives are earth, water, air. And it reaches towards the fire of the sun.

Our personal journey is similar. For some of us the mud may represent the emotional turmoil we so often find ourselves in. Some will call it the shadow, the neglected part of the psyche where whatever is not acceptable is relegated. Often our lifeforce has been locked away with the contents of the shadow, so like the roots of the lotus we need to draw up the nourishment, the energy, from below. The mud could also represent the collective unconscious; the deepest part of the psyche.

Of course to plant a lotus you have to get your hands dirty. It will only flourish when the roots are embedded in the mud. To your eyes the mud may look at first uninviting, even fearful. Most of us don't really want to stir up the mud. We hope that one day the water will be clear and calm, the sun will shine and all will be well. We certainly do need some days like that.

Unfortunately the mud usually contains not only nutrients but toxic waste. This stunts growth. We need to sift the mud, to filter it, to stir it up and separate out what is not natural to it.

Like plants, we seem to be designed to grow towards the light. Because of difficulties in the past it is as if we have grown towards the dark! When we were a seed beginning to grow the sun was obscured; our direction was not clear. We were often in shadows, often in coldness. We carry the memory of that inside, in our cell structure. Our growth depends on eliminating the old memories, clearing the sky, so the sap can flow again.

Our roots may be likened to our ancestral beginnings. Transpersonal work has shown that these connections are still alive deep in our psyche. Breathwork in particular is a method whereby ancient and personal shadow energy can be retrieved. Breathwork allows the sap to flow that circulates the nourishment. Our roots are our anchor too. Many recognise a need to be more earthed, to approach life and the journey with our feet more firmly earthed. Earthing is a prime background quality of ERC described in this book.

The sap carries the nutrients and carries away whatever needs to be eliminated. We might see our sap as the lifeforce energy that enables a connection between our conscious and unconscious, and between our mind, body and feelings.

The central plant stem could be likened to the central streaming of our core energy and the channels of energy that flow through and around our body. You may feel these energy flows activated and operating more strongly after deep emotional release work, and so can verify from personal experience that the ancients got it right in charting these meridian flows.

This central energy flow and the centres of energy — chakras, represented in our analogy perhaps by the buds — transfer the subtle energies that sustain us, as well as the emotional energy that needs to flow in order that we remain healthy.

The water through which the stems pass is traditionally likened to our personal unconscious. We know that in the pond there may be fish or snails, insects or waterbirds that live in and around the water. They may attack the stem. Certainly we know that at the beginning of our healing journey our own unconscious seems to hold some hazards. Full health for the lotus depends on the water as the link between the air and the mud.

The leaves of the lotus are quite like our senses. They have the possibility in good conditions to open wide and receive light and gather energy and transform it into a usable form. Have some of our leaves long ago learned to stay closed, denying us much new energy?

The lotus flower is the most visible part for those who do not look below the water. Perhaps the colour, shape and perfume are like our ability to express and create. Often though we have beliefs — learned in childhood — that it is not safe to open too wide, and you may feel yourself still at the bud stage.

The flower is a symbol of the energy centres through the body (the chakras) but, like our development in general, these centres only open fully in ideal conditions. This opening takes place in the air. The air itself is a vital part of nourishment which also conveys the warmth of the sun. The air represents the visible, conscious part of life dependent, of course, on the underwater world and the mud, which are unseen to the casual observer.

The sun may be like our sense of the divine because it draws us on and sustains us. It is often hidden by many clouds yet remains as the primary source of life. Whether you are working on personal healing or spiritual development in your journey you are aiming towards the sun. Many believe it possible to move towards the light and warmth without regard for what is below (the unconscious). In ERC we aim to clear the clouds and stir up the mud so impurities can be sifted out.

Some contemporary personal development approaches work to reinforce the hope that if you simply, repeatedly, focus on the air and the sun you will grow. However, most of us have obstructions in the stem, so we cannot draw up enough nourishment. We have a bud but it cannot mature. And we may sense that only when it matures — when we deal with the past hurts — can it open and really take in the energy of the sun and air and express what we are. Sometimes we try to peel open the petals. Sometimes we choose to believe someone else can help us recognise our perfume, our colours, our beautiful shapes. But as you use the healing methods, face the inner difficulties, stay awake to discern what is real for you, the inner work that leads to maturity unfolds naturally.

Definitions of ERC

Work with ERC will open up and free trapped energy. It allows the individual's 'inner healer' to do the work. Using the ERC modalities allows this inner healer to emerge through gaining trust in your own process of healing and trust in your own unconscious. Gradually you can prove to yourself that there is an inner force that reveals, with its own logic, what you need to remember, feel, release or integrate. As trust grows in this natural movement towards wholeness so your healing journey will accelerate.

A part of the healing journey involves realising that the ego cannot direct the healing process — it must step aside. Naturally your ego has learned to protect you from emotional pain. It is usually active in blocking out unpleasant memories and feelings and it always struggles to retain an idealised self-image. At some stage you have to consciously confront this automatic process.

It is unnerving to accept that you may have feelings inside which could affect you strongly. Experiencing these feelings may mean you need to 'fall apart' for a while. It can also be unnerving to realise that you are much more than you were told as a child, that there is so much more to you than the ego.

In our culture it is considered normal to stay home or remain inactive for a time if you are physically sick or injured. However, if you are going through a time of dealing with emotional sickness or emotional injuries, society is much less tolerant. We usually expect of ourselves — and others expect us — to do our inner healing work, and then quickly get back to normal and be completely focussed. But returning to the usual (old) way of functioning could force you to deny the new self. Emotional healing takes time and rest just as physical healing does.

Much ERC work begins with your reactions, hurts, disappointments and frustrations with your current life. Discovering the links between what affects you strongly now and past difficulties is very important. ERC is about improving your self-love, maturing your relationships, connecting with and improving your home environment, reclaiming your sensuality and sexuality, orienting your career from within and bonding with family — if that is a true impulse. To achieve these major outer changes, we usually work to clear the unfinished business from the past and release the blocked energy.

An initial aim of ERC is to become undefended — open to others and to your inner world. This may be a prerequisite for becoming 'transparent to the divine'. To become undefended generally you may have to explore specific issues. Following the ERC programme outlined here will take you far along your healing journey. Professional support can also help you drop defences during counselling time, completely feel your blocked feelings, remember the past, allow its release and open to the new inner space that results.

Give yourself time to integrate the feeling of released energy and inner harmony. Take time to consider any outer life changes that may need to follow your insights.

The following is a summary of some concepts that form the background of ERC.

Inbuilt motivation

Everyone has an inbuilt interest in self-discovery but often this urge has been stifled by disappointment and trauma. Inner healing work allows it to re-emerge, forming the basis for further personal development.

Old ideals

ERC tends to turn upside-down the usual notions concerning what is 'appropriate' in your emotional life. Ideals such as being able to hold yourself together, hide your tears, hold your head up high despite overpowering feelings, or soldier-on despite a recognition of internal chaos, must all be allowed to wash away. Through this the old deadening ways of being moderate, toned down, keeping your energies manageable and denying yourself for the good of another can also be dropped.

The value of emotional first-aid

ERC can operate as emotional first-aid. It can also lead into therapy — a second level of aid — and inner work with professional support. ERC allows you to stop repressing your feelings and to start releasing the day-to-day frustrations and hurts. ERC helps you turn daily life into an ongoing adventure of self-discovery. Finally it prepares you to enter the deep healing work that addresses more directly early childhood and birthing trauma.

Trust in your own process of healing

The unconscious in each of us has its own timing and logic. Problems in inner work often arise from the ego dictating what ought to happen and when it should happen. I call this impatience. As you learn to trust the unconscious to reveal and release as it is ready, you begin to feel very safe with this work.

Why not just focus on the light?

Negative feelings and memories in the unconscious are active and have an enormous influence on how you make choices and live your life. Bringing them to consciousness is the first step in disempowering them. Positive qualities, feelings and memories in the unconscious tend to be inactive, or overshadowed, by the negative. Making them conscious empowers them to be part of your life. The expression of positive feelings and qualities reinforces their proper place as a background to your character.

You may need to find the light before confronting the dark. Many new therapies and personal development courses tend to ignore the 'dark' or shadow side of our natures and turn only toward the light — real or imagined. These approaches can raise our hopes but they rarely lead to balanced development. It is, of course, useful to arrive at recognising our value before facing a past or present in which we may not feel valued.

The link between therapy and spirituality

ERC solves the 'problem' of the differences and divisions between personal healing work and spiritual work. Any ERC investigation that is carried through with patience and deep awareness leads to a more subtle inner connection. This internal connection, whether it be with emotional, physical or psychic energy, is the prerequisite for genuine spiritual search.

Trust

The modalities in ERC practice and the journal questions in this book are arranged so that you can spend time developing self-trust, for example during the quiet journal times, before beginning confrontative work with yourself, a partner or a counsellor. This need to develop trust applies to all your inner work and should not be rushed.

Defences

Help from others and your own willingness will enable you to recognise your defence mechanisms. These reactions tend to come up at times of stronger feeling to protect us from both present or past hurts. Defences include denial, projection on to others, blame of others, continual argument about details, etc. They were developed for a purpose. If you work to drop defences you must be willing to feel what was being defended. Remember to be patient and gentle with yourself!

Traumas

Traumas are events so painful emotionally or physically that they have to be repressed from consciousness. They build up from womb to adulthood. What was too painful to feel is put aside (as a safety mechanism) and you experience a partial shut-down. When feelings are shut-down or repressed the material, which is now in the unconscious, can have a powerful effect on the psyche. It can lead to 'acting out' through delinquent behaviour in youths and neurosis in adults. It can make us lead lives that do not seem to be of our choosing.

Repression is an unconscious mechanism where thoughts, feelings and sensations are locked away from our usual consciousness. Everyone carries a large number of repressed memories. Repression takes place chemically in the brain through the production of endorphines which are morphine-like hormones that have a tranquillising effect. It also takes place electrically in the nervous system where our neurotransmitters can impede or enhance nerve signals. This repression is reflected in and supported by tight muscles and shallow breathing patterns.

If you cannot cope with, or need to hide, inner turmoil and feel a stigma attached to this, then you need support to recognise that it is actually your openness, your work against repression, that makes you so vulnerable. This vulnerability will be very helpful for your healing work. Your friends who seem so 'together' may actually be more hardened or more successfully repressed and less ready to grow.

Interpretation

Interpretation of your inner world and its symbols by another person blocks self-discovery and can foster dependency. You should never tell someone else what their healing process means and what their symbols mean. This can be difficult for counsellors who are used to giving feedback, and for your inner child which may want to be told what is wrong, what to do and what internal things mean. A more vital way to grow is through self-discovery. Realisation of your own meaning gives confidence and a sense of healthy independence. Arousing your interest in self-discovery is important on this journey.

Goals

It is good to spend some time clarifying the outcomes you desire from your inner healing work. There are questions in the book to help with this. Some of the likely positive outcomes that ERC brings include happiness, self-confidence and a discovery of intrinsic spiritual dimensions. Some outcomes may not be considered positive by those around you: assertiveness, vulnerability, a sense of freedom, unwillingness to 'cope' with the old stressful situations.

Inner witness

An inner witness is needed for healing work. This is a part of you that objectively watches and learns from each step. It marks the difference between processing and acting out or dumping your feelings. If you have extreme anger or hate you may feel frightened of losing this inner witness and being overwhelmed or allowing feelings to release in a destructive way. Usually we will not let ourselves drop to such deep levels of feeling without having support that we trust.

Projection

All counsellors and people with a willingness to support others must be sure they are comfortable with the range and depth of their own and another's emotions. They need to create and be part of a safe environment for the expression and release of feelings.

Support people need to be on guard against projecting their own needs, conflicts or fears on to others. Projection occurs when someone is not in touch with their own deep feelings and in fact presumes that the feelings are actually coming from the outside.

Patience is also essential; a support person's expectations can intrude on a process that has its own timing.

Reactions

Angry or violent outbursts and over-the-top reactions come from the backlog of unfelt feelings stored away. To help resolve an emotional crisis in the present you search through the emotional layers underneath the anger to locate the original hurts.

To come to a new emotional freedom you feel and express these underlying hurts through processing.

Processing

Processing involves triggering an encounter with incomplete emotions in a structured, safe and supportive environment. Anger, hurts and frustrations are given full expression and released. This mobilises any feelings that have become stuck, and will save you having to act it out unconsciously throughout your life. Deep processing is usually done with a trained counsellor, but you can begin to focus on and experience your feelings more deeply. The exercises and information in this book will help you find out for yourself where you may have become stuck and to gain some release.

The boundaries between the processing room work and actions in real life need to be clear. If you allow yourself to be 'full-on' in a processing session you will not be tempted to act-out in your daily life.

Breathing and movement

Self-exploration with ERC approaches works to reverse old shallow breathing patterns. As children we reduced breath to reduce feelings and contain our excitement. As we grow up it remains the same and, in some cases, it gets worse. ERC helps the breathing to expand again. The expansion can bring a release of tightly held emotions and energies.

Your inner healing work also frees restricted sound and movement patterns. Bioenergetics is a great help here (see page 152). Many of us have learned to hold back our real voice and to censor our words. We have learned a few set postures and movements and tend to remain limited within these.

The links between body, mind and feeling

Your body, mind and feelings work as a whole. What you do not let yourself feel or express becomes stuck and feels negative. It turns into muscular tension or armouring (see page 152). These unexpressed feelings then drive your destructive thoughts and can lead to disruptive or destructive actions.

Underneath any physical tension and pain are emotions held in and emotional pain. When the physical is focused on, and the breath opened, you can feel again and, ideally, express the underlying emotions. Then the body softens, and you can return to a state of relaxation and happiness.

Underneath layers of anger and frustration is usually much sadness and hurt. ERC takes you down to an awareness under the layers and helps you contact the hurt. Under the hurt is the original state of love and tenderness.

The hurt inner child

The 'hurt inner child' consists of old feelings and behaviour patterns learned in childhood. Unlike many therapeutic approaches which allow the inner child a permanent position, ERC works to bring separation from this unauthentic part. It is only a hang-over from the childhood lack of fulfilment. In general ERC aims to integrate all real aspects of ourselves except this inner child which actually needs to be minimised. The power of the wounded, needy, inner child is reduced by repeatedly allowing ourselves to feel (in a safe, supported space) what the child did not feel or blocked off from feeling fully.

As children we often had to turn our anger inwards. We often felt ourselves to blame for parental shortcomings. All our attempts to be self-destructive or take on blame must eventually be released by being expressed outwardly in a symbolic way in the privacy of our room or with support in the processing room. The energy and feelings of anger and frustration that have accompanied the blame must flow out symbolically towards those who originally controlled us, blamed us or implied that we were guilty of causing family upsets.

Come home to your body

Since all healing takes place in the body, ERC helps you become deeply connected to the sensation of your body. It is usually in early childhood that the mind/body split begins. Through your inner work the split can be healed. Somewhere along your healing journey you will realise why you had to become a 'head' person; you feel all the reasons that kept you in a fantasy world of thought. After this process you can 'reincarnate', come home again, and allow your conscious awareness to be alive in your body. This is a hugely exciting step and brings profound positive changes in the way you perceive and interact with the world.

Group work

Once you have begun your journey of self-discovery you may find that group work is often more effective in bringing to the surface the old issues that need to be cleared. Groups create a strong atmosphere of permission to feel, cry and express. Trust develops, and the work of others can trigger, inspire and accelerate your own work. Groups answer the newly emerging urgent need for peers who can understand and support your inner life. They help you learn to live out the new insights and ways of being, and are valuable for checking reality.

Some theory on trauma and repression

The chain of hurts, disappointments, unfulfilled needs and hidden trauma usually goes back through time. Negative traits and experiences are passed on from generation to generation, from grandparents to parents to children, and then if there is no healing work, on to the next generation. This section is an overview of the chain of hurts. It explores why almost everyone needs some personal growth work.

Trauma is physical, emotional or spiritual wounding, of a serious magnitude, that cannot be integrated into the system. Hurts and disappointments are carried near the surface of consciousness but if they continue to be compounded over time they become a trauma.

How do hurts and trauma build up? A mother's emotional state at the time of giving birth will depend on her own birth and childhood relationships with her parents — her personal history — as well as her present relationship with the child's father. This emotional state, plus her health and her environment, will influence the womb environment and the birth. The womb will be 'friendly' or 'hostile'. A hostile womb is one that can be toxic or flooded by negative emotional energy. This can also create trauma. The birth will flow or may be obstructed in some way depending on biological and emotional influences of the mother. A difficult birth can set the pattern for the baby's way of experiencing and responding to the world.

Immediately after the birth there are strong needs for physical care, touch, emotional warmth, recognition and unconditional acceptance. Few of us receive full satisfaction of these needs. Deprived need leads to painful sensations and feelings.

This deprivation is imprinted in our mind or memory. The part of us we call the 'hurt inner child' grows out of this imprint. During adulthood it can never be satisfied in the 'here and now' because it is formed from this old imprint. It wants what the child wanted from parents. The imprints of further deprivation are recorded together with the original load.

Experiencing too much of this deprived need, for too long, overloads the system and results in trauma. Of course, sudden hostile and violent actions also cause trauma.

Trauma is 'gated' or disconnected from consciousness; we call this repression. Gating or repression requires constant energy. Researchers have found that it leads to a build up of stress hormones, an increase in body temperature and increased brain cell activity. These symptoms also emerge when repressed material breaks through from the unconscious in emotional release or breathwork sessions. Faulty gating leads to a kind of nervous breakdown when the repressed material breaks through. Good defences and strong repression can make someone appear mentally healthy.

The breakthrough of repressed material can motivate a person to explore therapeutic help. ERC and breathwork are therapies that cooperate with, and encourage, the 'opening of the gates' which is a surrender to feeling repressed material. There are some psychological approaches that actually strengthen the gates, and so help a person feel superficially better and have a stronger ego.

Repression results in so many limits! It can lead to a feeling of depression arising from some feeling or memory being pushed out of consciousness. Repression gives us the ability to ignore vast amounts of trauma — a life-saving ability for young ones. But for adults it sets limits on our ability to feel our emotions, creates a tightened or 'armoured' body and eventually compromises our health. It brings physiological changes and a disconnection between body, mind and feelings. This disconnection leads to forgetting our spiritual nature and who we really are.

There are two main levels of repression: the first is in the brain and the second is through our behaviour.

A defence mechanisn in the brain may be electrical whereby neurotransmitters impede or enhance signals, or chemical, where endorphin (like morphine) is produced to tranquillise your feelings. Long-term 'stress' uses up the natural tranquilliser and then a person may turn to prescriptions for painkillers or tranquillisers to deaden repressed emotions.

If there is an overload or leakage of repressed material the secondary defences — learned behaviours — come into play.

There are literally hundreds of behaviour patterns that you can use to defend yourself from feelings. Examples are:
- dumping — where the cause is outside you;
- rationalising — thinking your way out of suffering;
- reacting — sulking, tantrums, explosions and implosions;
- blaming — finding present causes for the old suffering;
- projecting — this happens unconsciously, we see what is inside as outside;
- armouring — muscles tighten, leading to a close-down of energy flow and feelings.

Most of these patterns are learned in childhood and form the 'character' of the hurt inner child. They are developed or refined as we mature physically but they keep us immature emotionally.

These behaviours help to either hold in or release the overload of emotional energy that comes from the past. They set our personality. A neurotic personality is frequently an attempt to solve the old pain through current behaviour. This never works for long. At best it may seem like a band-aid.

When you are ready you can find support to feel again, express and release the old needs, and the stored, hidden memories. For this trust and some understanding is needed; trust and understanding of the natural, inbuilt healing mechanisms. Trust allows you to drop the secondary defences of your behaviour. Understanding shows you that it is not madness to begin to actively suffer. What was too much for the baby or child is not too much for the adult.

Active, conscious suffering of the held-in past is the key to real healing. Active suffering is agreeing to be in touch with feelings — present and past — and to express them in wholehearted sobbing, raging or hating. All ERC processes require the agreement to some level of this active suffering. Through this we move into active enjoying, a new pleasure in being alive and being who we really are.

ERC methods are ideal for allowing this to happen safely. This book is designed to help you clarify what is happening in your emotional life and help you gain insights into any aspects of your psyche that may need further work. Working with the questions in this book will help you discover more about yourself. This discovery brings the rewards of new clarity, renewed energy, clearer motivation and supports your resolve to further your healing journey.

No one pretends that the journey is easy. The process of opening the inner gates and healing the past hurts and traumas is very challenging and at times may require skilled support. Once gates are open they cannot be closed as completely as before. This is good if you wish to journey on but challenging if you wish to stay the same. The release required for your complete healing may be much more than you suspected at first. Opening to your unconscious and allowing it to heal may take more time and courage than you imagined. The time frame for deep healing is never known ahead of time.

Positive character changes can be dramatic as you pursue the healing journey. Most people report feeling more forceful, more alive and more certain of their direction. Living in-between the repressed world and the free world can sometimes be uncomfortable at first. The new taste for freedom may make the old routine of daily life seem less and less acceptable. However, a deeper level of self-discovery will usually inspire us to continue on our journey!

There are countless rewards for this healing work. Many new personal and spiritual dimensions open up to us. There is a reconnection between mind, body and feelings which brings the experience of wholeness and of harmony.

Many people experience improved health. Since there are fewer and fewer old blockages to consciousness, new levels of consciousness open up and we actually see the world around in a fresh, positive way. We begin to like changes instead of fearing them; we become more adaptable.

Our old secondary defences of neurotic behaviours are no

longer needed and we begin to relate to others in a straight-forward way. More energy is available for creativity, not just maintenance of our daily lives. With this extra energy our spirituality can be felt as a here and now experience.

A life-long journey that begins with the quest to escape from inner pain brings us into a realm of new meaning, pur-pose, satisfaction and a deep security. It allows us to create the life we really want and to find new ways of expressing love and care. It releases us from the 'chain of hurts', allows us to drop defences and become vulnerable, or open, to a more subtle lifeforce within. Through our own experience we also learn how to support others in their exploration. Being able to do this allows us to contribute directly to the ongoing healing work that is so vital in the world at this time.

2

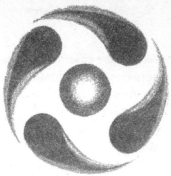

Leaving the Base Station
THE FIRST STEPS OF INDIVIDUAL HEALING

All of us are children in need;
and we spend a lifetime hiding that fact.

Arthur Janov from *The Feeling Child* (1977)

Recognising the hurt inner child

This chapter explores the Introvert Stage of the healing journey when you deal with releasing the past in order to grow into a fulfilled future. A vital component of this stage is dealing with the hurt inner child.

The wounded inner child is an immature part of each person's psychology. It is a collection of negative influences from the past. It is perhaps the strongest limit on growth towards wholeness. Recognising that you have a hurt inner child, understanding how this part is formed and how it can be healed, and working with it in day-to-day life, is one of the major steps in allowing us to really grow up.

A large part of your interest in undertaking the healing journey is surely to become an empowered, creative adult. Healing the hurt inner child part supports this and there are many other positive outcomes. One major outcome is the new freedom from fear. This includes the sorts of fears that we learned as children, for example: fear of authority, fear of not being special, fear of women, fear of men, fear of being real.

Allowing yourself to feel loved and the ability to express love can be reclaimed but first it is necessary to feel and release the emotional hurts that block your love. This process allows you to identify your true feelings and to experience them more fully. You also become able to feel and follow excitement. Most of us had to dampen our aliveness and excitement as children to gain approval. As adults, the renewed ability to feel excited not only adds much colour to our lives but, at a deeper level of our psyche, it leads us to recognise our purpose.

Healing the inner child also enables wholehearted reconnection with sexuality. The energies of love and sexuality can be reunited within. This is only possible after a release of any old fears relating to sexuality that were learnt in the early years.

Generally healing the hurt inner child brings a renewal of energy and gives us access to a deep well of creativity. It brings freedom from the nagging internal parental voices — known as the inner critic. This leads to feeling real self-love. Self-love and a sense of freedom from the inner critic are both crucial supports in moving forward with confidence on our path in life.

The child/adult concept

Emotional Release Counselling distinguishes between the happy, fulfilled spontaneous aspects of childhood — which are fully integrated into us — and the hurt inner child. These positive parts, often called the playful, or magical child, are over-shadowed by the hurt inner child. The negative child is like a separate identity made up of unfelt, or blocked, feelings. The playful part is the real you.

The hurt inner child is actually an accumulation of un-resolved, unmet needs, incompleted feelings (feelings blocked off, but held in suspension and repressed) and learned behaviour patterns that were adaptations to the early environment. So this hurt inner child exists in us emotionally and behaviourally. The child/adult concept is about the way this past of ours has an impact on the present. It reveals the truth that 'time does not heal', but simply allows feelings to be pushed out of sight.

Young children do not use their minds to understand hurts; they just feel the lacks, the disappointments, the longings, the traumas. Then they build up a defence against these hurts — a survival mechanism. Children begin by blaming themselves for the lacks. They often carry the load of their parents' short-comings. This stops genuine self-esteem from developing. It leads to a few basic negative beliefs about self and these carry on into adulthood and sabotage life.

The child's guilt at not being good enough to be loved, seen, held or appreciated has strong undercurrents of resent-ment. Anger is the reaction to being hurt. These undercurrents of resentment and anger have to be held down. If they were expressed this would compound the child's problem. Thus an idealised self-image develops. The 'bad' is pushed down and forms the 'shadow'. A life-long struggle develops between the ideal and the real (even though the real is often forgotten).

When a past hurt is triggered by some incident in the present all this unconscious resentment wells up. This often happens in an 'over-the-top' way so that the reaction is out-of-proportion to the event.

To heal and release your emotions you must go back through layers of reaction:
• False forgiveness
• Rationalisation, intellectual understanding
• Feeling reactions — anger, resentment, hate, and so on (the real feelings)
• The hurt of not being loved, seen, held or appreciated.

After releasing this hurt there is no longer any need to be defensive. It becomes possible to connect with your own inner resources and this connection opens you to a quiet, tender inner space.

Your ongoing task is to recognise actions which represent 'trying to win' or 'trying to get it right'. This action will keep you tied to the past and your idealised self-image. You also need to recognise the main survival or defence mechanisms you, as a child, developed — isolation, self-blame, living only in your head or disowning your real self — and work free of them.

The big change that comes from this healing work is a change in loving. We move from expecting love to being able to love. Love is now able to flow out. From feeling empty and needy, we grow towards feeling abundant and generous.

Healing the hurt inner child can be a long process with surprising insights and sudden progressions in self-understanding. It can release much energy and enrich your sense of really being a creative adult. A simple way to begin to understand the child/adult concept as a reality within you is with journal writing.

Keeping a journal is discussed in detail in chapter 3 (pages 47–63) but you can start right now by finding a blank book and trying out a few preliminary exercises. You may like to keep this as a private activity, using the writing as a way of opening up your memory and allowing your inner self to communicate with your outer self. It can be even more enriching to share your journal work with a partner, friend or colleague who is also interested in the healing journey.

JOURNAL QUESTIONS
Reviewing my past

This journal exercise will help you build a fuller picture of the influences from your past — especially childhood — on the present time. This fuller picture may include some previously unrecognised issues or emotional reactions which are still alive and kicking deep inside. Becoming aware of them and acknowledging them will be a first step in working free.

Think back to when you lived with your parents. Write as much as you can on these questions:
- What was the best thing about your mother?
- What was the best thing about your father?
- What did you dislike about your mother?
- What did you dislike about your father?
- What did you need from your mother?
- What did you need from your father?
- What made you most angry about how your parents were with each other?
- What reactions towards your parents do you still feel?
- What reactions towards your sisters and brothers do you still feel?
- Do you recognise any way that unfulfilled needs from your childhood appear in your relationships now?
  Review your writing and note how you feel now.

◆

A 40-year-old woman writes about the effect of the hurt inner child on her family life:

It came as a shock to see how the hurt inner child's need for a happy family back then had crippled honesty and freedom and sharing in our family group now. I found that I had been running myself ragged, attempting to arrange events where I could be with my children and my partner with his children. None of them wanted to spend time with each other. Nobody seemed concerned except me. I began to see that my inner child's need for a happy family was pressuring everybody.

After I felt the child's pain of never having the happy family she wanted, the relationship between us all changed. Each person felt free to have the kind of relationship they wanted with the others and the tension in the group eased. The adult part of me gave everyone permission to have the kind of relationship with each other that they truly wanted. I learned that what I — the adult — really wanted was, not so much a 'happy' family, but a functional family. I wanted one in which feelings could be expressed and issues addressed and talked about rather than kept silent, so as not to upset mum's need for a happy family.

Childhood trauma

Children want to be loved exclusively and without limit. Their ideal scenario would be 24-hour parental attention! They come out into the world expecting parents to live up to the womb experience; to be totally nurturing and present every hour of the day. Children don't want to share with anyone. Some of my clients say they expected their parents to be representatives of God. I imagine they would have been satisfied with continual, mature love and warmth, but most of us missed out on this, in some areas at least. The capacity for giving this unconditional love is rare. Most parents are still partly occupied with making up for the lacks in their own lives, and with keeping house and paying the rent or mortgage.

The pain of an unfulfilled relationship between parents and children can cloud over strong original impulses of love.

Many ERC clients report reliving the agony of being full of love and not having it received or understood. Our sense of unfulfilment, the hunger for mature love and warmth, often becomes the ground that begins a search to find completion within.

Throughout most of life we remain unaware of this longing; it is unconscious. However, we also unconsciously try to remedy the situation in later years. We sometimes even reproduce a situation similar to the child's in order to try to correct it — to get it right this time. This is done with job situations and particularly when seeking partners and friends.

Beginning the journal work and process work of the healing journey can reveal how we have actually chosen our partners because they have a characteristic in common with a parent who has fallen short in offering real mature love. Often we exaggerate and provoke this characteristic so that the child in us can try again to make the changes it wants. This never works!

When our inner work of releasing the past from mind, heart and body returns us to a natural state, unencumbered by a lifetime of disappointments and repressed hurt, our impulses of love, tenderness and compassion re-emerge. We no longer expect to struggle as the child did. These feelings can now guide us towards a new and deeply rewarding lifestyle; more determined by the aims of giving and sharing than by old needs to get and keep.

The happy, fulfilled aspects of childhood have been integrated into us. The capacity for joy and spontaneity is alive in us as adults but it is eclipsed or sabotaged by the hurt child part.

One of the glories of emotional release work is that it breaks the chain of negative conditioning. For example, my father was shaped in his ability to relate to me by his father. My ability to relate to my son has been extended or stunted by the modelling of my father. Generation after generation, the repressed feelings of hurt, and the inner and outer disconnection these feelings engender, are passed on. A son looks to his father for love and support. He doesn't see that while his father seems to be moving ahead in life, emotionally his father has his back turned. In many respects, adults are looking back longingly — consciously or unconsciously — towards their own parents.

Each child looks towards their mother and father as models for encouragement, shelter and love. The emotional maturity of the parent determines their ability to give. If by some stroke of good luck they are mature and do meet the child's need, the child too grows to become emotionally mature and able to give. But most children are still trying to complete something in their inner development. Very few truly leave childhood behind. Young adults may appear to mature and make their mark in the world but the motivation and the longing remains the same: to get what was not forthcoming to the child. Since the child's time has passed, this partly explains why so few worldly achievements give lasting satisfaction.

When children have been beaten, abused, emotionally or physically brutalised in some way, the tender, altruistic impulses are even more deeply buried. They are locked away under feelings of unfulfilment and hurt, and these in turn are beneath layers of rage and hate. Most children learn to suppress both the hurts and the anger at being hurt because they need to live in hope that, if they are very 'good', they might finally get what they want.

Childhood hurts are among the initial issues that emerge in early stages of the healing journey. People discover why they have struggled for so many years to attain something which has in fact always eluded them. They learn why they have stuck with a project or a relationship that did not bring satisfaction, and why they struggled for years trying, they finally realise, to get what the 'child' wanted. Negative belief systems are exposed. The beliefs of the child have become beliefs for the adult, and many of these actually rationalise the lack of fulfilment or satisfaction in life.

Working with bioenergetics and dance, and tuning in to the sensations of the body, reveal the child's posture in us. It is usually one of contraction and slumping. Moving through the pain of childhood allows the freed body to find a new adult posture; one of strength and expansion (similar to an untrammelled toddler).

ERC gradually allows these layers of repressed emotion and the memories that go with them, to return to consciousness, ready for release. It is possible to access life-determining traumas from all ages. The journal questions in this book can begin this process. The next steps will happen if you are really willing to feel and express now what was too painful to feel and too dangerous to express back then.

In separating from the child part you begin to recognise the adult steps life is calling you towards. Promise the hurt part that it will be given more time to feel and release. This is the best way to really care for it. Healing the hurt inner child is an ongoing process and it may take some time.

Each new freedom and insight is swiftly tested. There can be a tension between the old conditioned way of living and the new freedom. The style of life set up by the hurt inner child feels constrictive to the newly emerging adult. You also begin to find that the rewards of healing the child's pain and moving towards adult fulfilment do not seem to have a limit. Gradually notice how you become less 'prickly' and reactive to those people you may have been reactive to in the past.

Fears in life that originated from childhood experience are diminished as they are worked through and released. Without ever directly setting out to achieve it, you will discover that life has become fuller and richer and freer. This sense of well-being becomes the foundation for further spiritual work.

There are many approaches to understanding and working with the inner child in contemporary psychology and counselling. Some are more effective than others. Beware of approaches that tell you to love the inner child. Although this sounds good and comforting, it is like inviting a neurotic and immature part of us to take pride of place in our psyche. For those of you who really want to mature it is imperative that the child's pain be felt totally, expressed and released. This may take some time. It may seem to require more than you feel capable of. It may shatter your illusions about yourself and your life. But, as long as you do not force inner work before you feel ready or allow yourself to be pushed by others, it is a real and safe way to become fully adult at last.

Healing the hurt inner child comes through processing, bringing emotions to the fore, re-experiencing and releasing the longing and the hurt of the crying child. We have to re-experience the acute pain we once suffered but pushed out of sight. It then turns into a healthy 'growing pain'. The hidden hurt flows away and there is less bitterness, tension, anxiety and frustration within. There is less of this child part.

Free of this wounded inner child we may discover a simplicity, a spontaneity, a joyfulness that indeed seems child-like. We might even call it our child part, but it is really us. The needy, wounded (and very strongly sabotaging) inner child is not a genuine part of us. It must be separated from in order for us to integrate and live out our positive potential.

Processing with the child/adult concept

What reactions truly belong to us as adults? What inner states are responses to the current situations of our lives, and which ones come from past conditioning? Which moments in my relationship belong to me, and in which ones am I propelled by imprints from past relationships?

As your inner work progresses it clearly exposes the inner child. This child frequently runs your life. Look within honestly and you may see, with horror, that you have been driven by this child which denies you autonomy. You will find a lot of freedom when you come to know the child and catch it at its tricks — using you to struggle for what it wanted. Acknowledging and feeling the hurts from the past will eliminate the unconscious pressures that drive you to set up new hurts in the present. Feeling the depths of the past needs will free you of their stranglehold on present fulfilment.

These same needs that may have been asleep under the surface, or well managed in our lives, can be powerfully triggered as you read this book or begin to ponder and face the truth of your life. Having support to clear the needs gives you the energy and psychic freedom to be creative and fulfilled now!

People in the helping professions will often find these inner needs triggered by all their giving. When they are able to heal the old needs and find new fulfilment their giving becomes truly enriching. They are then truly able to help without depleting themselves or projecting their unconscious needs on to those they are supporting.

Most children develop some emotional survival or defence mechanisms. The strategy that often leaves us with chronically

low self-esteem is to take on the blame for parents' shortcomings. If a young child recognised that parents just simply could
not give them what they need emotionally it would be too
much to bear. So many survive by presuming that the fault is
in themselves and if they just keep trying to change then the
parent will love them fully.

Other defences can be seen in a need to put oneself down
before others can, or modifying everything that is said so that
it will be agreeable to others. Each of us must discover our
own defences against feeling parental shortcomings so that we
can stop recreating the childhood patterns.

JOURNAL EXERCISE
Does my past set my present?

This exercise helps draw out parallells between your present
reactions and hurts and those you had as a child. It can reveal
why some events in your current life are so upsetting and why
you sometimes compromise your real self in the struggle to
make up for the past.

- Start a new page in your journal. Rule a line down the
  middle.
- Head the left side THEN, head the right side NOW.

1 **Right Column — NOW:**
- Think of a current problem or emotional hurt — write it
  down briefly.
- Write down any reactions to the hurt (e.g., anger, resent-
  ment).
- Write down any reasons or rationalisations or blame you
  carry around the issue.
- Take a moment to let yourself feel under all this — close
  your eyes, take a few breaths, tune in to your feelings.
- If you stay with that you will find under it all the hurt of not
  being loved recognised or appreciated in some way.
  Describe this in simple words.

2 **Left column — THEN:**
- With what you have just written in mind, re-evaluate your
  relationship with your parents when you were a child. Take

time to think and feel it, allowing any images or memories to float up into your mind. Summarise your relationship with your parents.

- Write about any attempts to forgive them.
- Write about your effort as a child to understand the reasons behind your relationship with them.
- Give time to knowing how you really felt about them under all this — summarise this.
- What was the main hurt you carried from that relationship with your parents? Write this down in simple words.

3 **Compare the hurts in each column.**

4 **Rule a line across the page and write across both columns:**
- What are the similarities between your parents then and the issues and people causing you hurt now?
- What is your hurt child trying to make up for, prove or get? Note this.
- Note how this child part has been trying to do the same thing in your life now.
- What was the survival or defence mechanism the child developed? Are you now good at it?
- What new steps or aims do you need to form to be free of the inner child's ways?

Goals for the emerging adult

Affirmations and goal setting for personal development are often considered a useful aspect of some New Age approaches to growth. It may be true that positive thinking has a beneficial short-term effect, but beware of artificially glossing over inner turmoil, or lack of self-esteem, with wonderful sounding affirmations. An affirmation may make you feel good during the moments you are thinking of it, but unless it has grown organically out of inner healing processes it really has no lasting power. Copying an affirmation from a book or using another's affirmations without deep pondering is also of questionable value.

It is important to ponder, meditate, search within and find the right place within, or the right attitude of surrender, from which to set goals instead of making lists and promises to yourself. Remember 'the road to hell is paved with good intentions', and the journey of inner growth and exploration can be wrongly directed by signposts of wishful thinking. These signposts, or promises to oneself, are usually erected by the ego for self-calming purposes. They also protect you from exploring right to the rock bottom of your truth; a truth that may have many challenging aspects.

It is vital that goals, wishes, intentions, steps, new directions are indeed set by the adult you, not the child. The child part, of course, has its own old agenda and narrow goals. Following these will lead to emotional regression and greater emotional dependency on others. But how can you know the difference?

If the focus of your wishes is to gain something from the outside, be suspicious! If your goals centre around discovering more inner resources you can proceed confidently. If your intentions are simple and straightforward, not complicated, they are more likely to come from you, the adult.

Other attitudes also indicate the input of the child part: hoping to win, the need to do something perfectly, fear of emptiness or being alone, plans that will create great struggle. An adult can be open to a range of outcomes and is interested to learn from mistakes. Adults are ready to face unfamiliar states of emptiness and can enjoy being alone. An adult certainly has to put an effort into their inner and outer life, but if there is a continual struggle you can be sure the inner child is lurking in the background.

Beyond the hurt inner child: empowering the creative adult

In the early stages of your healing journey you have to deal in depth with the destructive, negative and limited beliefs of the hurt inner child. At a certain stage it is essential to support the creativity of the adult who begins to emerge, free of the old conditioning. This emerging adult self is still learning how it wants to live and what it is like not to automatically react as the child did. It is important then to explore some ways of further empowering this new stage.

Maintaining a clear adult energy in yourself depends on regularly taking the small everyday steps to make your outer life more in harmony with the new energy within. It also depends on finally giving up the hope that the hurt inner child will get what it wants. You have to come to a decision that the adult in you, not the child, will emerge victorious.

When you don't follow through with your new directions the energy released through inner work actually becomes available to the child part again — you regress. Following through with adult steps entails taking risks and possibly making changes in career, relationships, hobbies and creative expression.

Regression also takes place when you let your energy become blocked. This can occur simply when you revert to old habits — usually old habits of being contained and being 'less than we are'. Regular physical, emotional, mental and spiritual exercises are useful for staying adult and clear.

As you move into the Extrovert Stage of your healing journey, you are more able to give. You have achieved some of the healing and growth of the Introvert Stage and have learned to give to yourself. Living with this new attitude of giving rather than always needing is very empowering. If you notice any negative reactions to the call to give you can use this as the trigger for further clearing and healing work.

One of the final steps in personal healing is the authentic expression of the lifeforce in creative, constructive ways that bring benefit and well-being to you, to your family and to your community. We need to search for our individual authentic expression. It can be a small, simple, everyday expression, or a really grand one.

Eventually you will hear a call from inside. The call is experienced differently for each of us, and is heard at different times. It is a call to express your adult self, the skills gained from your journey, and the released energy out in the world. You may need ongoing help to really listen for this call, and dare to follow it.

This calling can be recognised by the special, deep excitement that it arouses. This excitement comes each time you follow your call to contribute to the world. Also, following your excitement can lead to recognising how to contribute.

It works both ways! Learning to distinguish adult excitement and the child's excitement is vital. The child feels excitement when it is hopeful of having its old needs met at last. The adult feels excitement at being alive and following directions from the inner world.

Some projects or careers will be life-giving for a while, then it will be time to move on, to face new challenges, learn more about yourself in new ways, find strengths in other areas. Resisting this natural change can be caused by the child's imprints, and resisting can trigger the child's attitudes to life and growth.

However, a creative adult sees change as a chance to make a fresh start. Each fresh start brings the chance to make your life more fulfilling, and out of that fulfilment find new resources for contributing. The hurt inner child usually views change as a threat.

The creative adult is often empowered by discovering and leaving behind the limiting beliefs that have been gathered through life. Sometimes, after considerable basic work on the child's hurts, discovering these beliefs can be a simple process of pondering and discernment.

One belief that many of us hold is that there is a limit to self-discovery, that we can go just so far with personal growth. Seeing obstacles and discovering new aspects of the self are insights which bring much energy to the creative adult, and are often themselves the creative stimulus. The adult may need support at times to reconnect with the inner self that knows there is no limit.

Regular personal development work will continue to clear the old material normally brought to consciousness by your psyche and by triggers around you. The ego is often looking for the time when inner work will be over; when we will be 'perfect'. The inner child may impose its ingrained belief that the need for further healing work is another sign of failure. Ongoing connection with a healing group can be a support in sorting this out.

Creative adults thrive with the companionship and modelling of others. Among those who journey a new sense of community can develop and it is vital that we nurture it. Networks of inspiring support remind us of the journey and the many ways that the fruits of the journey can be expressed in the world. One adult step is to take responsibility for creating this inspiration through contact with other travellers.

Creative adults who have listened deeply to themselves find that they can listen and share more deeply with others. There is a feeling of greater depth in relationships and more connection when we share ourselves with friends. Empowerment comes from sharing true feelings, the visions of the future, and taking risks in revealing our real selves.

Quiet times — usually when you are alone in stillness and silence — are often a necessity for clear discernment. These are times when you should become physically and mentally neutral to listen to the inner self. This needs practice. Only when the outer doing self relaxes for a while, when the ego shuts down for a moment, can the inner call be heard and the nourishment from within be felt. It can be a challenge to include these times in a daily routine.

After extensive practice, this meditation time will connect you in a wordless way with the divine energy inside that is always flowing. Further work on old imprints (on the Lower Self) is more effective as you gain access to your Higher Self.

The creative adult can live and love with increasing pleasure. While the ability to serve and support others grows, there is a letting go of elements in our lives that really do not work, that are chronically struggle-filled and unpleasurable.

This growth in pleasure usually leads to a sense of gratitude for being alive and for the journey we have undertaken. We feel gratitude towards those who have helped us grow: our models, our teachers, and the pioneers whose lives created the methods we use. It is a support for the adult to find ways to express this gratitude. Lack of gratitude occurs when the child's neediness is predominant and it is a sign that more inner healing work would be profitable.

Unexpected artistic and creative activities can emerge for the empowered adult who is undertaking the healing journey. These talents may be discovered through drawing, dancing, journal writing, work with dreams, sitting in silence, and through following a spiritual practice that brings harmony to body, mind and feelings.

When we have glimpsed who we really are it becomes

painful to regress. But it does happen and many find there is a great temptation to be disheartened by a temporary return to the old confused, helpless, needy child state. Confronting these changes — which can sometimes feel quite extreme — is really a new challenge. The answer always involves our responsibility to work on ourselves. This call to inner work will probably go on forever. This is journeying.

So, when we are finally freed of the child's compulsion, we will no longer cry out to be loved by the parent, but will seek a future, a partner with the aim of finding the maturity we really want. In not demanding to be loved, we can begin to find self-love — resources of love within ourselves. As we love ourselves more we mature.

Perhaps the most vital aspect for our journey is that in not demanding to be loved as a child we will be deeply willing to love. We will seek love in a different way: by giving it, instead of unconsciously expecting it! When we have dealt with the hurt inner child's pain we become able to love maturely, and a benign chain reaction can begin.

The adult who is constantly engaging in the inner work of the healing journey reclaims passion for life and is free to give attention wholeheartedly to the task at hand. There is a sense of wonder in more areas of life. Life is lived creatively. This creative energy illuminates your impressions of the world around you. It enhances the nourishing qualities of inner work such as meditation. This energy brings wonder and fulfilment to your daily activities.

3

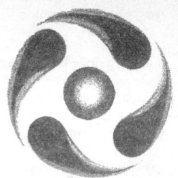

Gathering the Explorer's Gear
NEW METHODS FOR HEALING AND DISCOVERY

Affairs and business will drag on forever,
So lay them down and practise now the Dharma.
If you think tomorrow is the time to practise,
Suddenly you find that life has slipped away.
Who can tell when death will come?

Milarepa the Buddhist Poet-Saint, from
The Hundred Thousand Songs of Milarepa
Vol. One Trans. Garma C. C. Chang (1989)

The methods of inner healing work that have been developed as part of Emotional Release Counselling can be used individually, with a group or with a trained facilitator. This chapter outlines the methods you can use individually at home for self-discovery and self-healing, and gives you many exercises to focus and develop your quest.

The aim in the following pages is to introduce dynamic methods that will empower the early stages of your healing journey. As an explorer, your equipment will include journalling, music and drawing, symbol work through dreamwork and sandplay, relaxation and meditation.

Journalling

Keeping a personal journal or diary devoted to the inner world is a simple first step in examining your life. It will help you see the ups and downs of emotion and motivation.

Journal writing begins to separate you from the whirlpool of feelings, desires and directions. It helps you perceive contradictions and confusion more clearly. Your dialogue with yourself in a journal begins to show that there is more than your conscious intentions at work in your life.

Often re-reading a journal entry after a period of time makes it possible to see the threads of unconscious impulses that are really directing you. As these impulses become more conscious you gain more choice about what you are doing, how you are relating and where you are going with your life.

Journal writing is a process. This writing comes from your realisation in the moment; it is a very 'now' process. It includes your thoughts and feelings, what you find within your body, what you find within your energy and the energy field around you. Journal entries can explore changes through time, for example daily and weekly reviews. To deepen the content of journal writing, be open to more than just recording. Be open to movement in your feelings, to new understanding and new insights at any stage.

When the writing process is really alive you can perceive subtle mood changes as you write. The light of your attention stimulates the unconscious to reveal buried feelings, beliefs and attitudes, and your self-understanding will grow.

One aim of journal work is to encourage your intellect to add its knowing by ordering and linking functions to the experience of the body and feelings. This is especially useful after a very intense period of emotional healing. The mind can bring integration to our emotional exploration. It links up insights and emotional experiences with intellect. Journal writing focuses the mind to:

- sort out what is going on inside us — hear all the aspects;
- record what we observe — insights, opposing and harmonious realisations, decisions, intentions;
- review where we have been — to bring perspective to the issues of our personal growth;
- resolve present problems;
- clarify future directions — to identify where our interest and excitement lie.

Journals are also places to record dreams for later work. In working with dreams you discover messages from your unconscious about the way you live your life. These messages can also be recorded for future review. Journals can support a sense of journeying with the symbols of your unconscious.

Writing in a journal is a way of giving yourself inner space. It is like an inner counsellor; in a journal you can talk with parts of your psyche, and this can bring a therapeutic benefit.

Journals are private so you can be truthful. Uncensored, honest writing will help you become more sincere and to face things that your ego may normally defend against. It is important to be clear about the privacy of your journal.

As a tool for reflection the journal helps you deal with reactions and prepares you for important and clear sharing with others. Relationship difficulties and your reactions to them can sometimes be clarified through journal work before confrontation with partners.

Journals allow your vulnerable and poetic side to emerge (most of us normally hide these aspects). And finally, journals create reflection time to re-assess your life's direction — to review the journey rather than merely to deal with the inevitable problems.

Journalling and self-observation

Journal writing is, of course, preceded by observing yourself — your outer life events and your inner life reactions, responses, moods, insights, aims and intentions. The practice of self-observation is essential to collect data on who you really are instead of who you presume you are, or wish yourself to be. It is the act of noticing and recording 'what is'.

Often we fall into a habit of trying to change ourselves, to be better people, to strive for an idealised image, so that we do not really know ourselves. This becomes obvious when some unconscious impulse leaps out from within unexpectedly — some anger, some hurtful words, some unexpected empathy. It is this lack of self-knowledge that allows some of us to drive ourselves into states of great tension or exhaustion. It means we may go through life without access to the full depths of our feelings and our ability to touch something higher.

Writing down your inner and outer experiences in a journal becomes an aid to self-observation; and self-observation becomes the forerunner to meaningful journalling. The two go together, supporting each other and supporting you in the adventure of self-discovery.

There are risks which follow on from self-knowledge: self-judgment, self-criticism, trying to change what is seen, rejection of what is seen! The great spiritual teachers as well as leaders in the personal growth field seem to agree on the principle of working to accept what is revealed in self-exploration. If you see that in fact there is a hurt inner child controlling your responses to the world, that you are not really free and 'adult', you may at first feel a bit depressed and angry about the past. The healing journey methods will help you work through all this.

Right from the beginning, we are advised to continue self-observation no matter what it reveals. Krishnamurti, a well-known twentieth-century philosopher, encouraged seekers to practise self-observation until it became like a flame that burnt away the untruth. Another spiritual teacher who reintroduced much of the ancient wisdom into our times, G. I. Gurdjieff, saw self-observation as the central inner effort at early stages of development, and cautioned against confusing self-observation with analysis or attempts at analysis.

Even as you ponder on something you have seen, you run the risk of not seeing the next moment. This act of self-observation, of gathering self-knowledge, is one of the strong linking points between personal growth work and the great traditions of developing consciousness.

The journal will be a record of your ups and downs, your emotional highs and lows, your sensitive and dull times. It will reveal how much you change from day to day, minute to minute. The journal will help strengthen a more objective part that can stand in front of your inner truth and begin to make clear decisions and turn your life in a definite positive direction.

Finding confusion and contradiction within can be painful, but it is a small price to pay for release from aimlessness, meaninglessness and chronic emotional suffering. The excitement of having a life of journeying is the reward. The journal work becomes a recorded trail of where you have been. This trail proves that you are moving forward in some way. It reveals the patterns of your inner life and helps set you free.

Some hints for journalling

Describe inner and outer events, processes and insights. As you write, remain in touch with your body, your feelings and the energy of the mind (especially any intent to change the truth).

Watch for a sense of deeper layers of meaning and feeling. Allow yourself to open to and resonate with them.

Clarify each experience. If you need to write a lot on a particular subject do so. Give time to each part of the experience. Give time to finding the exact words — this clarifies the experience.

Record changes. Describe the new, higher, or more flowing energy that may emerge as you engage in self-exploration.

Watch for and record the emergence of new wishes, new aims for your inner work. Only record affirmations that have come from deep within yourself.

Record inner child/adult insights and any new light on your basic behaviour patterns.

Acknowledge anything that you kept hidden in group work or from your counsellor.

Describe your dreams and draw them. Write down insights from Gestalt role-play work (see page 75).

Research symbols from dreams, fantasies and mandalas. Find traditional meanings of symbols and colours (see Further Reading page 184).

Include mandalas and drawings (see page 70 for examples).

Counsel yourself. Imagine the challenging questions a counsellor might ask you about your inner and outer life and answer these. For example:

- What has been hidden or unclear until now?
- Exactly how is my childhood imprint active in my life now?
- Have I blamed anyone? Do I need to make changes here?
- What are the risks in moving forward and claiming my true self?
- Who would be upset by my growth?

◆

Journal writing about a recent period in my life
45-year-old man

The crossroad of deciding to follow my inner truth and marry and begin doing counselling work with people is based on a new truth in my life. This is not an attitude of waiting for permission from the outside but of giving myself to the direction that comes from the inside. I sense in myself a flow of inner peace, new energy, lack of restriction, of no longer being trapped, but, as well, a lingering sense of guilt or shame. It's like I've done what I needed to do to give myself to love and life and I am made to feel guilty for it. I always say to myself, 'You should not have done that'. It's like giving birth to myself and feeling an atmosphere of not being okay. Deep down I know I had to make the changes. It feels right when making the decision — the after time tries to pull it down. I remember the insight from my childhood, 'I will be punished for showing initiative, excitement and energy'.

I notice in myself a new sense of body harmony. I still wonder if I drink to fill the emptiness, the hole, but I am not sure what the hole is — maybe it is just feeling the feelings — grief, or sadness or excitement. Drinking feels like a NO to full aliveness. I know that I am better without it but I still do it!

I sense a change around money — less of a panic, more of a sense of flow and letting it be there for use, for movement, for people rather than a static build up for security, something to hoard for a rainy day. My security is in the now, the energy of the moment, the time and believing that will happen when I give myself to it.

Important note

These journal exercises are arranged in a specific order to support the gradual deepening of your inner exploration. I suggest you work with each one over a period of time in the order they are presented.

JOURNAL EXERCISE
Where should my emotional healing begin?

Begin with this simple journal exercise to help pinpoint areas
in the past and present that may need deeper investigation. It
will give you a starting place to identify more clearly where
inner work is needed, where old emotions may be blocked.

Write whatever comes into your mind about these areas/
times of your life:

• Your siblings and your place in the family.
• Your birth — family stories or family circumstances at that
  time.
• Your mother's emotional state while pregnant with you.
  If possible ask your parents about this.
• Where you lived from birth to teens.
• Your childhood relationship with your mother.
• Your childhood relationship with your father.
• Any other main carers.
• Your religious upbringing.
• Any physical, sexual or emotional difficulties or abuse to
  you in your childhood.
• Your memories of your childhood.
• The main expectations on you in childhood.
• The disappointments about yourself in childhood and
  adolescence.

When you have written about each, before continuing, re-
read and ask yourself how you feel about the past now and
how you really felt about the past then.

JOURNAL EXERCISE
The chart of inner and outer events

This review exercise will take some time. Afterwards you may
have a clearer sense of the times in your life that have not been
resolved or integrated.

Divide a large page into three columns.
Column 1: Write notes on what you know or remember of
the main outer events of your life. Start with birth, then your

earliest memories of being a toddler, childhood, adolescence, leaving school, earliest sexual experiences, romances, first jobs, major relationships, deaths of people close to you, and so on.
Column 2: Write down the approximate dates.
Column 3: Try to comment on how you felt inside about each event. You may also include any special, more vivid or conscious moments that stood out from the rest of your experience. List here any knowledge you may have about how you closed down or opened up your inner world. Include the most powerfully positive and the most traumatic, negative experiences.

1 Outer events	2 Date	3 Inner events

JOURNAL EXERCISE
Overview of this stage of the inner journey

Think about your life now. This exercise is designed to give a broad overview of many aspects of your inner growth now. Take time to ponder each question. Try not to censor any answers — be interested in what your unconscious presents first. Review what you have written after a break and see where you need to focus for the next step. People I have worked with often get a surprise during this exercise as new areas of exploration and focus emerge.

• Take time to relax and come home to yourself.
• Write briefly on each of these questions:

Issues and concerns
• What are the main issues that incline you towards inner healing work?
• How do you feel about those issues now?
• Can you feel any progression in your accessing, understanding and resolving of them?
• What current situations are you most negative about?
• What current situations are you most positive about?

Emotions

- What do you suspect is the main feeling still buried in you?
- Are you aware of a time-lag between your feeling and its expression?
- What causes the delay or, alternatively, what hastens the expression of your feelings?
- What are your main fears or anxieties?
- How have you progressed with these feelings?
- What is the main fear waiting to be faced?

Emotional release work

- What are you most afraid of in processing your blocked feelings?
- What is your main motivation in doing some inner work now?

The wounded inner child

- Are you really able to feel the 'child'?
- How often do you catch that unfulfilled 'child' in charge?
- What are the risks, or adult steps, you need to take in light of your discoveries about the wounded inner child?

Your body

- Have there been any changes in your health since you began your search for emotional healing?
- In what way is your awareness growing around:
  - muscular armouring
  - energy flows/blockages
  - emotional flows/blockages
  - lifeforce and chakras
  - left/right differences
  - your attitude to your body?

Resistance to growth

- What do you most resist in your growth?
- What is your main way of resisting?
- What does it feel like to break through a resistance?

Relationships

- What do you hide in relationships?

- Do you feel a growth in ability to share from your heart?
  - with one special person
  - with a group
  - in everyday relations
  - with yourself?

Sexuality

- What is the most unsatisfactory part of your sexual expression?
- What is the most deeply fulfilling aspect?
- What are you really longing for?
- What is your main fear?

Spirituality

- What has been the effect of your inner search on your spirituality?
- Are there any recent changes in your understanding of spiritual life?

Aims

- List your main outer life aims.
- List your main inner life aims.

Summary

- What emotions has this exercise evoked?

JOURNAL EXERCISE
The daily review

This simple exercise invites you to choose a week and for every day of that week to spend a period of time in the late evening reviewing the day and writing down your observations. You can continue after the week, but it is better to select specific lengths of time to do the exercise — aiming at forever is really too much for the part of us that resists self-awareness.

Write down brief notes on your day under these headings:
- Major outer events.
- Main reactions to these events.
- Main moods you were aware of in yourself.
- What things really took priority?

- Were there any moments of helping or relating well with others?
- What did you do for yourself today?
- In retrospect, what seems to have been the main aim of your day?

Now consider tomorrow:

- Do you have any specific intentions for yourself, any main aims?
- Is there an area of your inner world you would like to observe more?

JOURNAL EXERCISE
The whole cast has their say

There are many parts to your personality. You have learned many roles. It is as if the cast of a large, popular stage show gives a performance every day. This exercise helps you acknowledge the various voices, sort them out, and begin to discern what the 'real' you is like.

Take a specific day and review the events in the evening. You are going to write a review from several different points of view. Imagine you are each of the characters below. As you write and picture yourself as these characters, let your body change and take a posture that goes with each:

- A very critical High Court judge.
- A laid-back beachcomber lying in the sun.
- A quiet monk or nun who lives alone in the mountains.
- As your mother.
- As your father.
- As the person you most admire.

Read over what you have written:

- Write down how you feel now.
- Which view is the most familiar?
- Which is most realistic?
- Which are pure observation and which are really criticisms?

Reflect on what you have just written, then write down an intention to know yourself without criticism.

JOURNAL EXERCISE WITH THE PAYOFF CHART
What is stopping me?

This is a challenging exercise and it can help you find out why you seem to get stuck at some point in your inner growth, in relationships, or in getting what you want in life. It can help you recognise why you so often do not let your energy be free and flowing. It can help you free up some lifeforce and release contraction held in the body. It uses the energy of insight which can be strong but is usually short-lived.

We are directed and motivated by pleasure. This exercise can show you how you derive something pleasurable or in some way positive out of how you are or from your situation — even if this seems to be negative or unsatisfactory on the surface. New insights will come if you recognise that you must get something positive out of your present state of affairs, or the real motivation to change would be there! There must be a plus in your present stuck state, no matter how ridiculous that may seem. Somewhere, usually hidden from view, is the payoff for staying the same!

- Set out the four columns described below.
- Tune in to your body, feelings and energy.
- Think deeply about the questions, visualising the real situations in your life and how you would like them to be.
- Allow yourself to write without censoring.
- Allow any feelings to be alive.

Column 1   *What Do I Want?*
Describe the problem you cannot come to terms with or feel stuck in.

Column 2   *What Blocks Me?*
a. Simply write all the things you can think of.
b. Visualise the blocked energy or events as flowing again.
c. Where/when did your energy and pleasure get blocked?
d. What was the original moment in your past (childhood) when you acted in a similar way?
e. Who have you blamed for being or feeling blocked in achieving your aims?

Column 3   *What's The Payoff For Staying Stuck?*

a. Write down everything that you do get out of maintaining the present situation. You may need some courage to own what you get out of being stuck; it is your payoff.
  • Watch for subtle energy movement within.
  • Note that hanging on to the problem or the victim stance is one way of staying special.
b. List who gets this 'positive outcome': the inner child or the adult?
c. Is there anyone that you want to come and rescue you?
d. Can you identify the roundabout way you have been getting pleasure or something positive from staying stuck?

Column 4   *What Is My New Wish?*

a. Make a new wish or form an intention that does not rely on others to be fulfilled. It should accept the principle of getting pleasure, satisfaction or fulfilment directly.
b. Write down two or three practical ways to carry this out.
c. Note how your energy feels now. Check if your body is holding down any lifeforce now. Note this, does it need to move or dance or take action right now?

◆

Sample exercise — What is stopping me?

A 36-year-old man writes in his journal

Column 1

I want to be more alive.

Column 2

a. My wife will not like the things I do. There's too much work to do anyway.
b. I'd leave the lawns and gardens and give more time to my pottery.
c. When I agreed to put in the new gardens for her.
d. I always had to do what pleased my mother. I wanted her to be happy.
e. I have blamed my wife, kids and parents' expectations.

Column 3

I don't want to own this, but I think I get a happier wife. I'm doing what she wants. But even as I write I know that she also wants me to be more alive (especially in bed!) I'm deadening myself to please her, but I do not actually please either of us at a deep level! Wow! I should have said no to those new gardens and actually told her that I want to do more with the clay.

Column 4

It sounds selfish, but I'm going to clear out half the shed and get some clay, so I can actually do what I want, when I want. And from now on we are paying the kid next door to mow the lawns. My main wish is to share with my wife what I really want to do and ask her to help me follow through. I can feel some excitement even now. Tomorrow morning I'm going to the craft shop.

ADVANCED JOURNAL EXERCISE
Why does my journey seem to be going in circles?

This exercise is designed to help you discover new ways forward. It is relevant for people who have been doing inner healing work for some time.

- Take time to ponder these questions. Relax, close your eyes and open to a deeper level within that can present you with answers.
- Then write as quickly as the thoughts flow. Don't stop to be accurate; let the writing tumble out.

1 Is there a deep memory or feeling that you know about but consciously dread; and therefore it limits deeper inner exploration?

2 Do you suspect that there is an unconscious memory or feeling that you are not ready to face?

3 Could the problem be an outer-life one rather than an inner world one? What changes in your outer life are you avoiding? What steps or actions — that you already know you need to take — have you put on hold?

4 What risks or challenges, connected with living out of the next stage of your life's journey, have you decided not to deal with?

5 Is there someone in your life that you react to regularly — bringing you into a state of regression — that you need to separate from?

6 Do you fear or resist separating from (abandoning or being disloyal to) your 'hurt inner child'?

7 Is there a strong here and now reason to stay very together that prevents you releasing blocked energies?

8 Are you afraid of your rage? Look inside for any hidden rage, hate or resentment that may be lurking there, no matter how unacceptable it is. What is holding the anger in doing to you?

9 Explore the inner child's beliefs about hope. Is there a basic hopelessness that seems to belong to you?

10 What are the main dangers in being powerfully alive, in living with pleasure and having fulfilment? List them all. What protection or safety are you secretly getting from a stuck state?

- Re-read your answers, looking for linking threads, and summarise the points to address in your future work.
- Do you need to make arrangements to get support in exploring more deeply now?

JOURNAL EXERCISE
What activities really give me life?

Could it be that each of us has a job, career, activity or purpose that is just right for us? Can you name a job which would bring you fulfilment, energy and excitement? Would this activity change as you develop? Could it be that what was the perfect job for you at age 25 no longer fits at 35 years or 45 years? Is it possible to earn a living from what you really want to do? Do you still hope for this?

Ponder these questions and write your response.

1 What was the main thing I struggled for as a child? Am I in any way still doing this through my job now?

2 What activities really excite me? Do not limit your answers to money-making things.

3 Describe what you get out of your present job.

4 What arts or crafts do you love or are you drawn towards?

5 Do you have any daydreams about careers or activities?

6 Is your present job a final one, or a stepping-stone towards finding one that is congruent with the real you?

7 If there were no outer constraints — such as supporting
 yourself or a family — what activities would you love to do
 each day? List several steps to help you begin to bring
 together your inner and outer demands.

VISUALISATION AND
JOURNALLING EXERCISE
Listening to creativity

Part one

Spend time allowing your imagination some freedom. Read
the following notes or better still have someone read them to
you slowly as you lie down and relax.

'Imagine yourself as having unlimited energy and strength.
You are on this planet for a purpose. Your body is very
strong and alive. This aliveness is wanting to express itself
through you. It wants to be used. Imagine you have enough
money to do anything at all. There is nothing limiting
you. So far in life you may have been striving to solve the
money problem, but just for now visualise your wealth as
unlimited.

'Visualise the special contribution your energy could
make to everyone on earth. Let images come to your mind
of the special things that your talent could create. Let
images come to your mind of two specific projects you
would like to do. They may be connected with your career,
or something you could build, invent or research. These are
things your energy would love to be involved in. They will
bring you great fulfilment.'

Part two

- Write down what your imagination suggested for these two
  projects. Try not to limit it by practical concerns.
- Consider what would be the starting point for each project.
- Now write down the main practical blocks to arriving at
  the starting points.
- Is there a compromise that may enable the project to
  become a reality?

JOURNAL EXERCISE
The people in my life

This worksheet will help you sort out relationships, reactions and problems with the people around you. It will help you pinpoint the source of difficulties such as continually being triggered into anger, grief or withdrawal. The aim is to identify when a problem comes from the other person and when it is in you. This exercise should help you to realise that you need to speak out about some relationships. The exercise on pages 64–65 was done by a 45-year-old man.

Music and drawing

Music

Music can soothe, annoy, or enliven us. Certain songs or sounds may bring out our shadow side and others may open us to a higher part. Musical vibrations can relax or wake up the body. We also use music to encourage the heart to open and release its load. Music supports powerful catharsis of old, repressed anger and hate, as well as inviting surrender into the tender, essential levels of being.

On page 186 there is a list of music organised around the main emotional moods. This music can be used as a supportive background for individual self-exploration and for group and professional situations.

Drawing

It is amazing how many people think they have virtually no ability to express subtle or powerful inner states through drawing. Most adults stop developing their expression through line and colour way before adulthood. However, I have found that with a little prompting we can all go past these perceived barriers in ourselves.

Much pleasure and integration comes through abstract expression of music and feelings with crayons, paints and pencils. I have enjoyed guiding many workshop participants to a rediscovery of their creativity and affinity for colour. Creativity and skill in drawing can be developed and greatly enjoyed. It is never too late!

JOURNAL EXERCISE
The people in my life

Person	Their colour	Their shape	Animal like them
Partner	Pink & orange		Dove
Ex-partner	Blue/grey		Fearful rabbit
Father	Watery grey		Weak deer
Mother	Scarlet		Jellyfish
Child — son	Emerald		Proud lion
Child — daughter	Light blue & gold		Strong dolphin
Sister	Purple		1000 ants
Brother	—		—
Grandmother — mother's mother	Silver & pink		Peacock
Grandfather — father's father	Flesh colour		Pig
Boss	—		—
Best friend	See partner		
Worst enemy	None		

Their big problem	What I would like to say to them	How I feel about them
Love too much.	This is it! Together for the rest of our lives.	Gratitude, love attraction.
Won't feel, rationalise.	Stand on your own two feet.	Regret, relief, burden.
Won't grow up.	It's not too late to be a father.	I try not to feel.
Gives in all the time.	You can do it.	Care and distance.
Thinks the world owes him. Afraid of the world.	You are both special and precious — a gift to me.	Love, amazement and much joy. Also grief at separation.
Too busy. Needy.	Slow down. Listen to me.	Care but distance.
—	—	Wish you existed.
Superior to everyone.	What about me?	I've lost you.
Self-important.	—	Glad you're gone.
—	—	—

MUSIC AND DRAWING EXERCISE
Surrender to music and free expression

Arrange a time when you are alone at home. Take the phone off the hook. Choose about five pieces of music that you like (or that stimulate a reaction). Choose music that can touch off and support these feelings:
- tenderness
- anger and an impulse towards catharsis
- grief, sadness, loss
- powerfully alive lifeforce
- wholeness, spiritual fulfilment
- letting go
- stillness
- movement and celebration.

See page 186 for suggestions about music.
- Organise a large drawing book and a good selection of crayons. Place them ready beside you on the floor (carpeted is best).

- Play each piece of music. Play it loud. Lie down and surrender yourself to it.
- Focus on being 'at home' in your body. Do not try to think about the music or the exercise. Let your ears open and eyes close.
- After each piece of music sit up and immediately draw. Just watch and see what colours you pick — try not to plan it! See what lines and shapes want to be expressed. Many people find difficulty doing this at first, but report that they quickly get better at allowing something within (not their mind) to guide the drawing.
- There is no special outcome intended from this exercise, other than helping you free your expression and surrender.
- If you like the drawings keep them.
- As you give yourself time to do this exercise the connection with your inner self grows.
- You may begin to notice some subtle emotional states that the music stimulates or reveals.
- Write in your journal about any emotions touched by the music.

DRAWING EXERCISE
Exploring your state with line, colour and movement

This process will open you to a deeper impression of yourself.

Drawing
- Place crayons and a large blank pad in front of you.
- Start at the top of the page.
- Close your eyes.
- Feel inside, listen to your state: the feelings and energy.
- Open your eyes. Choose the right colour from your crayons for how you feel now.
- Open your breath and draw a line that corresponds to your state. Really look at it.
- Feel — is it exactly right?
- If it is not right draw again, or choose another colour. Try again, see if you can get closer to representing the inner state.
- Since you have begun to tune in, there will be change.
- Keep going, drawing lines and assessing whether they reflect your feelings, until you reach the bottom of the page.
- Perhaps there is a word that goes with the lines? Let it come to you.
- Feel the energy with which you draw. Let the feelings continue to be in the energy, in the hand.
- Let the breath be open.
- Use the act of drawing to help you own exactly how you feel.
- Ask yourself: where is all this happening in me? (If the drawing looks wrong, turn the page and keep going.)
- Keep tuning in. Is the line heavy enough? Light enough?
- Let some sound that seems to express the line come out. What sound goes with the colour? Is it clear? Mixed up? Differentiated? Superimposed?
- Risk making the sounds to yourself that go with the drawing and your inner state.
- Is there one word for the picture of your inner state?

Movement

- Take the drawing to an open, clear space.
- Stand in front of it.
- Take three very full breaths and relax them out.
- Find the posture that goes with the drawing.
- Close your eyes now.
- Let some movement start now. Try not to control it. Let it change and grow.
- Let sound come too if it wants to.
- Let the movement increase and exaggerate, let it be tighter, faster, slower, more flowing — more of what it is! More rhythmic, more chaotic.
- Let your energy express itself totally. Let the sound grow. Put your whole body into it!
- When this feeling and expression takes full volume on every level it will change.

Surrender

- Surrender on to the floor. Think to yourself, 'This is how I am now. Can I surrender totally? Is there another degree of surrender possible?'
- There is nothing to do now. Let the breath be however it is.
- Open yourself to receive whatever comes from within. Let a colour, a word, an image or a memory come to you.
- Simply be with it for a while.
- When you are in touch, gently sit up.
- Don't analyse. Take time to record your experiences.

Mandalas and emotional release drawings

The term 'mandala' denotes the ritual or magic circle used in Lamaism and also in Tantric yoga as an aid to contemplation. C. G. Jung

Mandalas are drawings done after a period of ego surrender. They are traditionally drawn within, through and around a large circle. They may be expressions of, or from, a connection with your unconscious or with a higher consciousness. The drawing is not planned. It forms a bridge to a part deep inside you and can be used as an aid to contemplate your journey. In series they form a valuable map of the healing journey. Mandalas are outer expressions of inner processes; how they appear to others is irrelevant, you create them for yourself. Remember your drawing skills are not being tested.

The circle on a large blank page marks off a sacred space for the unconscious to express itself. Studies by a Jungian analyst show that it is more therapeutic to draw in a circle rather than a square or rectangle.

It is ideal to draw a mandala immediately after periods of inner healing work before discussing your feelings or insights with anyone. The drawing should be done while the energy from the unconscious or transpersonal levels is still flowing strongly. Most people find that mandala drawing brings a deep feeling of completion to their counselling session or inward focussing time.

Time and attention should be given to the mandala work — the full attention! Don't let your interest start wandering or spreading out to others too soon. You can honour your inner work in this way. Honour the process — provide yourself with good large drawing books and a full range of crayons.

It is the unconscious that is revealing and recording itself. You offer your hand, your eyes and the crayons to be used. It should not be the conscious mind that draws because the mandala comes from beyond the ego. Do not interpret immediately — allow the energy experience to nourish you from the mandala. It has its own healing potential.

Never allow anyone to interpret your mandala for you. You may think you see important images or insights in another person's mandala, but you must let them do their own learning from it.

Mandalas seem to radiate meaning and energy for a long time. Open to this. Analysis and research on symbols and colours can come later. Spend time simply looking and watching for insights.

You may wish to display mandalas in your home in chronological order. Spend time contemplating their messages. Review your mandalas from time to time.

There is a difference between mandalas and emotional release drawings. The latter are part of a release process; we do them when we need to express particular feelings. Emotional

These two mandalas were drawn by a 48-year-old woman.

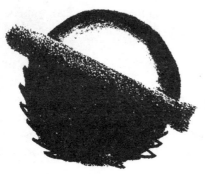

She writes:
This mandala shows my
blocked rage from an
abuse incident when I was
12 years old. The blocked
rage left me feeling 'I am
powerless and weak. I have
no rights or say in this.'
An insight came that
henceforth from that time,
I led a 'hazy existence' in
which I could not feel
much of my life. After working with this realisation I felt an
energy that was alive, vital and real.

This mandala shows my
expression of long held-in
rage around feeling
dominated and humiliated
in the past by older or
male persons in my life.
There was no doubt about
the use of the colours red
and black when it came
time to draw the
experience. At the end of
the session I felt brilliant
— very connected to my
power.

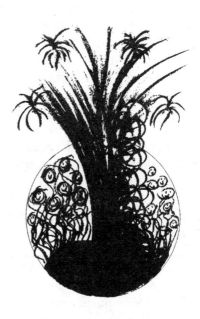

release drawings are usually not kept. They exist simply as a vehicle for expression. They may express anger, fear or sadness. They are used to help us get in touch within and to let something be completed.

REVIEW EXERCISE
What more can I learn from my mandalas?

- After a period of intensive inner work, spread out your drawings and mandalas.
- Which ones seem incomplete and could be extended off the page? Imagine what would be there, then allow it to be drawn, using extra paper.
- Look at the dark and the light colours and the strong and the faint lines. Consider the possible meaning of these variations.
- Ask yourself if the drawings are predominantly about: the inner child; deep feelings; the body; energy; the unconscious; the Spirit; special memories; current relationships.
- Look for repetition of: colours, themes, shapes, moods, symbols.
- Are there any clear divisions, splits, or strong connections in the drawings?
- Is there a progression, sequence or a transformation?
- Are the boundaries being broken? Is the energy contained? Unbounded? Outside? Inside?
- What were the main messages in them?
- What does the series say to you right now?
- Take some time to research any specific symbols.

Symbol work
Dreamwork

You can use everything in a dream. From dreams you can reintegrate your disowned personality. Every bit of each dream is yourself. If you really play it out fully it becomes part of you again, and instead of being more and more impoverished, you become richer and richer and richer. Fritz Perls

Exploring dreams is a useful technique for self-discovery and healing for several reasons. Although there are different types of dreams, different levels of seriousness, they can all provide helpful insights.

Dreamwork is a means of expanding our understanding of the symbols used by our unconscious to make itself known. Symbols contain or transmit much more than words. They work on an emotional level as well as having a positive effect on the body. Integrating dream symbols gives us our personal mythology and helps us understand the language of our unconscious, and to follow its directions.

Dreamwork helps us to resolve issues. The unconscious mind has a built-in mechanism for releasing the past and resolving conflicts. It tries to do this through dreams. Taking the time to work on a dream is a way of co-operating with your unconscious and speeding its healing work.

Some issues that may be presented through dreams include: current problems in your day-to-day life; deep fears that are surfacing from the past; re-emergence of disowned energies or characteristics; or birthing energies being released. Dreams also give clues about the direction of your spiritual evolution.

Dreamwork helps you recognise and integrate repressed traits or characteristics. For example, sexual dreams may be about coming into union with some inner aspect. In this case your reaction to the dream will give a clue to its meaning. A peaceful reaction would indicate a sense of completion but if you react with agitation or alarm there may be something to learn and work with.

Guidance for the direction of your inner work can sometimes be suggested in dreams. Many of us have had to put on hold what we really want to do in life, but this calling may still be alive deep inside. Your dreams may be the only time when these wants can surface. Dreams also may show you situations to be faced, or indicate new attitudes to what you have to face.

The inner world is perhaps the main topic of dreams. Dreamwork is a major support in opening to this inner world and accessing your inner energy.

Dreams should be treated seriously, even if they seem silly. Make no assumptions except that the dream makes sense.

It is often tempting to rush to analyse or ascribe meaning in a cognitive way. Sometimes we like to prove that our conscious mind is as smart as the unconscious! It is much more valuable to take a few moments more to integrate at an emotional level using the simple Gestalt method (see page 75).

Dreams can reveal the content of your unconscious: the wounded parts; repressed emotional material; positive undeveloped abilities; advice about your direction in life; and, of course, the voice of your spiritual self that is rarely heard in your waking state.

For dreamwork to yield its treasures, you must want to dream and want to remember the dreams especially the 'big' dreams. Every now and then, when you are going through a significant growth period or large-scale outer changes you may have a major dream. These are usually dreamt in your deepest sleep. Minor dreams are important too, and they hold much richness for day-to-day living.

It is good to go to bed with pen, journal, and access to light ready. Develop the habit of asking yourself, 'Have I dreamt?' as soon as you wake. Those who find that they never remember their dreams can explore their day-time fantasies in the same way that night-time dreams are worked.

Next write the dream or fantasy down. The writing is a way of making sure you remember as much as possible. It also helps you open up to the message. As you write, look for symbolic language. The important words will have a charge.

Drawing the dream images is also a way of letting the dream speak. While drawing or painting you are staying close to the unconscious, and perhaps some clues to the message of the dream will emerge.

Ask someone to listen to you retell the dream. As the telling proceeds you may suddenly hear words, phrases or descriptions of aspects of yourself that strike chords of recognition. This process can be quite exciting or sad. It is easy to be caught up in the story or the emotion but remember that inner listening as you speak is vital. The energy of the dream will be activated and this conscious expression helps resolve and integrate the dream. When this happens you will experience a shift of feelings and energy within the body.

Some dreams do not need to be worked on because they

achieve an energy shift and insight as they occur. Those of us who find the expression of anger difficult in our waking life can break through this fear in dream, and shout or kick and be very free in expression. After an active dream your nervous and muscular systems will be more relaxed, and your outlook should be more positive.

If the underlying message of a dream is important it will recur. We often have recurring dreams. The most common of these are to do with fear. Fear is the key feature of nightmares about being chased by monsters, gangsters, or in some way being threatened.

The ERC method of working with dreams, scary or 'normal' is to gestalt the dream using the simple questions and steps evolved from Fritz Perls' work. (see page 75). It is important to write down every symbol — animate and inanimate — that occurs in the dream. Sometimes if symbols appear to be contentious or in opposition to each other you can make up a dialogue between them, changing roles until resolution is achieved. If you appear in the dream yourself the other main symbols can set up a dialogue with you.

Gestalt dreamwork is a major part of Gestalt psychology. It was developed by Dr Fritz Perls and others in the USA during the 1960s and 1970s. The concept in Gestalt psychology that I find most useful states that an unresolved feeling, memory, attitude, energy, trait or quality will stand out and be in the foreground of the unconscious. Working with this notion to bring about release, resolution and integration means that the unresolved feeling recedes into the psychological background.

Aspects of yourself that are prominent in the foreground, though not recognised, are easily and often projected on to others. It is as though these aspects are coming towards you from the other. This projection of our unconscious also takes place in our dreams as we sleep. Our unresolved feelings are transferred to dream symbols.

A simple way to integrate or recognise the aspect of yourself that is in the foreground in the dream is to role-play it. Totally 'becoming' the dream symbol brings new awareness and integration. Hence to really understand dreams, or fantasies, fixations, or compulsive attractions, you simply play at being the thing. To effectively 'become' or 'gestalt' the symbol, you need to be relaxed, have awareness focussed in the body and allow movement, sound and expression.

DREAMWORK QUESTIONS
Gestalt method of understanding dreams

You can work alone with this exercise, or do it with a friend or counsellor, but do not ask anyone to analyse your dream. Avoid asking others to give you the answers. Growth will occur only if you make your own discoveries.

- Come home to your body, tune in to sensation, breath, heartbeat.
- Close your eyes. Take the part of the dream with most energy: the most vivid, best remembered, or most troubling part. Let the scene become clear in your mind. If working with another, describe the scene.
- Play all parts of the dream. For each symbol begin: 'I am a ...' Then describe:
  - your appearance,
  - what you are made of or what is inside you,
  - your actions or movements,
  - your function or purpose,
  - your intentions,
  - any special message.

Listen to your own voice if you are speaking aloud; feel the meaning resonating inside.

- Let yourself move and make sounds if they want to come. You can stand or take different postures if it helps to integrate the energy into the whole body.
- Never interpret another's dream or decide the meanings from your head.
- Allow the story to progress.
- Allow the dream symbols to dialogue with each other.
- Finish with a statement about the message of the dream.
- Write down your results and transformations. Draw a mandala or picture of the dream. Research symbols for the traditional meanings if you have more curiosity (see Further Reading, page 184).

Sandplay

Sandplay is an individual process although it is usually done in pairs — one person supporting, the other exploring — or with a trained counsellor. It is a useful tool for:

- resolving personal problems
- reclaiming forgotten qualities
- opening to inner guidance and direction
- expanding self-knowledge and personal mythology.

Sandplay is a way of translating the images in your mind into graphic expression, and it may help you discover previously unconscious thoughts, feelings and attitudes. It makes vague feelings more concrete and clarifies confusion. Things that may have been swirling around in your psyche can take definite, ordered shape, and through this reveal deeper meanings.

The process of sandplay is carried out by making a picture or story in a sand tray, drawing from a large array of miniature figures and objects. A single session may take fifteen minutes or it may take an hour or more — it is up to you. The figures chosen correspond with meanings in your unconscious, although sometimes you will choose figures which represent themes already in your conscious mind. Most often the connection between your unconscious and the chosen symbol will be revealed during the session.

You can start this way of exploring your inner world by collecting hundreds of figures. These will be easy to gather as you ask your children, your relatives and begin to scour opportunity shops, souvenir shops and toy shops.

Then when you have time to yourself, or are working with a friend or partner, you can start by looking at the figures which are lined up in categories on a shelf. As you look you may feel that some of them reach out to you. A strong feeling of either repulsion or attraction indicates that a symbol is obviously important in your psyche at the moment. Select the symbols that call out, and arrange them in the sandtray — a little like playing on the beach. You may not realise it at first but a symbol calls out to you because it resonates with something inside you. Alternatively, you may begin by playing with the sand, arranging it, heaping it into hills and valleys, rivers or coastlines.

The process is similar to working with dreams where the symbols are chosen or created by your own unconscious. In sandplay, the symbols are outside you, ready for your unconscious to project its meanings on to them. Your unconscious emotional state, if you allow it, shapes a landscape in the sand, selects the symbol figures and arranges them on the landscape.

Working with the sand and the symbols is a wonderful way of exploring your inner world. It is very non-threatening and potentially very revealing. Look at how you relate to each figure and how they are arranged in relation to each other. Sandplay often highlights aspects of yourself that remain hidden in a traditional counselling session.

It is tempting to look on sandplay as a bit of a lark at first and this is good because you will move into it more easily. It is an ideal technique for people who lack confidence in their verbal skills, or those who are unused to opening their thoughts and feelings to others. It is also useful for integrating and clarifying a period of intensive inner work. In group work, selection and arrangement of symbols — even if there is no sandtray available — is a good preparation for sharing your inner world more clearly and more deeply.

There are many categories of figures in a mature sandplay collection. The important categories to begin with are: mystical, religious, the sea, mechanical things, buildings, precious stones, household items, food, wild and domestic animals, nasty things (skulls, big black spiders, snakes, rats, skeletons), adults, children, babies, fantasy people, natural objects (rocks, gum nuts, branches, shells), symbols of war (soldiers, Indians, tanks, guns, jets), containers (boxes, fences), birds, jewels, transport, flowers, trees, bridges.

You should not ascribe set meanings to the symbols. Use the exercises in this book to discover your own unique meanings.

Background of sandplay

Sandplay itself originated in England with Margaret Lowenfeld who published her findings in 1935. Dora Kalff, a Jungian analyst, with the encouragement of Jung himself, studied with Lowenfeld in London, then returned to Switzerland to begin her practice with children. She used Jungian symbology and developed her own version of sandplay. She began with Jung's hypothesis that there is a fundamental drive toward wholeness and healing in the human psyche. It is reported that her patients made rapid and exciting progress. The same stages of healing in the psyche were observed when she worked with adults.

The difference between free play and sandplay is having a structured setting, a facilitator or support person, and a clear intention to understand yourself. The facilitator is actually an observer whose presence calls up an observer in yourself. You begin to understand what is happening inside because of this observing part. The sandplay will shine a light on the unconscious and its messages.

Using sandplay

While sandplay is a valid tool on its own for self-development, it becomes more powerful and effective when blended with Gestalt work and Emotional Release Counselling. The sand-tray can be used for the expansion and exploration of a specific crisis, the surfacing of an old hurt, or for acting out what is not acceptable in daily life. It can also give an overview of your present journey. This overview often acts as a reminder that your journey is a positive, life-affirming experience.

Through sandplay we can gather data about the unconscious self-image (e.g. 'I'm no good', 'It's no use being female!'). Many people realise they have disowned aspects of character or disowned energies, and often these energies have been labelled negative. Through the sandplay session any so-called negative energy can transform into a usable, creative force and be integrated.

After some training, we can all support others in sandplay, as long as the golden rules are observed:
• do not interpret another person's experience,
• allow any emotions that are triggered to be released.

There are no other rules apart from respect for the materials. The person who is exploring is always right in his or her choices and arrangements. The support person, although vital to the process, is neutral.

If you are a support person, try to drop all that you know

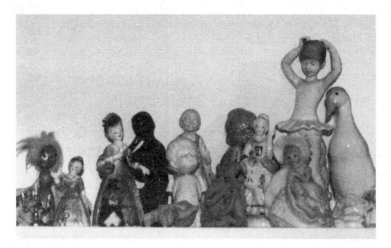

A typical sandplay symbol shelf. In a collection of hundreds of figurines, each one can be used to represent a feeling, person or event you may need to deal with.

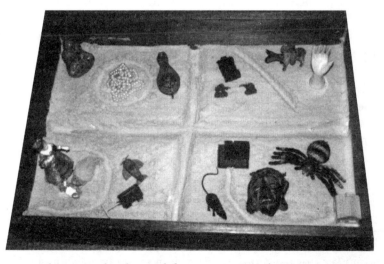

This example of a sandplay exercise Family Portraits *(see page 82) was created by a 40-year-old man. The lower left square represents 'You as a baby'; lower right shows 'You as a child; the upper right is 'The present'; and the upper left is 'The future'.*

about the person who is exploring. Be with them, physically and mentally, mostly silently. Watch the choice of objects and the way they are chosen. Be aware of the development of the story. Bring a presence, a focus, that will support the journey and the person's acting-out or telling of the story.

Try to recognise the symbolic level but never interpret, never tell the explorer what you think it is all about — even if it seems very clear to you. Realisations and connections are of no lasting use unless they come from within.

As all the symbols used represent energies within the explorer, help them consider the meanings they attach to the symbols as well as the possible traditional, collective meanings.

Watch and help them notice the placement of the objects. What is in the middle? What is at the edges? What dominates? What items are separated? What is buried? What is in water? What is on the hills? What is under attack?

While watching, supporters should keep track of their own personal reactions and assumptions, to avoid projecting their own story on to the explorer.

To complete the session, the explorer may tell the story. If emotions have been triggered by the process, go with them, encourage expression. Never make a connection for another. Always lead them indirectly until they realise something for themselves.

If appropriate, the explorer can write down the story of the sandplay. They can take a Polaroid photo of the sandtray to keep in their journal.

GESTALT EXERCISE WITH SANDPLAY SYMBOLS
'I am ...'

If you have a a particularly strong response to a figure in your sandplay story, or you suspect a deep symbolic meaning in a figure, you can deepen your exploration with this exercise. This gestalt work can also be used if there are only sand formations and no figures.

- Sit in front of the sandtray. Leave the symbol(s) in place.
- The support person asks the you:
  'What do you like/dislike about this figure?'
- The support person then says:

'I want you to become this figure for a little while. Feel yourself as it. Take a breath.

- Let your body change. Take the shape of the figure.
- What is it like?
- Tell me what you feel like?
- Describe yourself: How big? How little? Colours? Shapes? Energy?
- What do you want to do? What sound do you want to make?
- Take another breath. How do you move?
- What are you there for? What is your purpose?
- Do you have a message for … (explorer's name)'

Often the figure will symbolise some aspect of power or energy which you have ignored or buried. By role-playing the figure, you can become more 'yourself' and have access to the power or energy previously locked away.

◆

Gestalt role-play with sandplay symbols
Max, a 45-year-old man writes in his journal

BUTTERFLY: I am the part of Max that can find the beauty and growth in himself and others, sometimes in the most unusual places. I can find the 'spot of growth and beauty' amongst the ordinary, the ugly, the thorny, anywhere at all.

CRUCIFIX AND BROKEN JAR: I speak of transformation. I am like a bridge between the old superficial respectability values and the new appreciation of those parts represented by the symbols — the essence of any painful struggle is transformation. Everything is on its way to transformation — that's the message of Jesus. Brokenness is often the vehicle of this.

TURTLE: I am the turtle energy part of Max. I continue the growth that the butterfly finds — through gentle transformative process I keep the new life emerging. I especially show there is no need for comparison, the essence of my presence is uniqueness — through the return to the genuine 'mother energy' of the turtle that is compassion, acceptance and love, I give growth to the unique new, essence of Max.

GOLDEN BODY RECLINING: I am the new emerging energy of the long time ideal of the ability to read, reflect, grow in knowledge, watch less TV, drink less and really enjoy the alive energy to grow in pleasure, calmness and depth of life. I hope to thread through everything eventually to bring calmness and depth to all that is done.

FLOWER SET IN A CLEAR SOLID BLOCK: I represent new creativity that is going to come from inside — gradually as Max gets more used to inner work and is more skilled and open. I will become more obvious. I, too, am linked to the butterfly and I show the new growth through the new solidity gained from inner work.

SHELL: I represent the new openness and vulnerability that has happened through this journey.

GORILLA: I am the new energy of life that has come through emotional and physical healing — new strength from not seeing a parent in every person. I am the energy that your mother tried to knock out.

BUDDHA: I am the new universal value that Max is now in touch with the world beyond the narrow limits of institutions.

SANDPLAY EXPLORATION
Family portraits

This simple process focuses on family relationships and their possible link to the present.
- Divide a sandtray or a large page into four.
- Set out the sandtray or page like this:

4. The future	3. The present
1. You as a baby	2. You as a child

This arrangement corresponds with Elizabeth Kubler-Ross' discovery of the way the psyche works in drawings.
- Select sandplay objects to make four pictures about each period of your life beginning with you as a baby. The symbols are arranged in the four sections of the sandtray or on the page.
- Talk about each picture with a support person either while it is being created, or after.
- Note the main similarities and differences between the pictures and with life now, and talk about these.
- End with journal writing, focussing on the insights gained.

Relaxation

I have never met anyone who considered themselves to be relaxed enough. Relaxation is an important element in the healing journey. Being physically and emotionally neutral means you must let go the way you brace against the outer world. You also need to recognise and make conscious efforts to resist the eternal distraction of your revolving thoughts. Relaxation exercises can give you a taste for a new way of living.

Successful relaxation is essential for balanced inner growth. It involves:

- taking time to recognise the depths of your tension;
- finding methods to allow the tension to drop away;
- finding and releasing the underlying emotional causes of chronic tension.

Part of the aim of this book is to help you explore these three aspects. The following exercises can be worked on each day. They can take two minutes or sometimes half an hour. Be aware that exploring relaxation will inevitably draw your attention to tensions.

There are many simple ways of relaxing: taking a long hot bath, lying down with beautiful music, exchanging a massage. Often it is hard to break out of a cycle of busy activity. We have not been brought up to value or enjoy stillness, emptiness or silence. However these states are often our first glimpse of a way to live that is more pleasurable and more real than allowing ourselves to be driven by the old tensions and habits of compulsive doing.

Real spiritual life is born from states of relaxation and surrender. The body is our doorway to the inner life. Instead of battling with thoughts or distractions, simply turn awareness to the life of the body — over and over. These exercises are designed to help with that. Do we value ourselves enough to make daily efforts?

RELAXATION EXERCISE
Relaxation using visualisation

This is a sequence that uses both physical relaxation and visualisation to assist the body to let go, and assume its natural posture. Allow at least fifteen to twenty minutes for this relaxation. It is ideal to have these steps read out to you with a long pause between each step. The subtlety of the exercise depends on visualising, thinking the relaxation, rather than doing it. Doing allows the ego to become activated.

- Lie on your back on a carpeted floor with a firm cushion or paperback books under your head. Find a comfortable height so your chin is neither forced down or up to a level higher than your forehead.
- Your knees are bent with feet flat on the carpet.

1 Visualise your neck becoming free and expanding up towards the crown of your head.
2 Let the trunk be free to lengthen and widen, visualise this. Let it 'follow' the head as it moves up. Visualise or think this rather than 'doing'.
3 Connect with your chest and belly. Give them permission to let go now.
4 Visualise your shoulders opening out from each other. Allow your body to follow this image.
5 Tune into your belly. Is anything tight? Let go in the belly now.
6 Imagine your legs letting go from the hips, as if the joints were becoming softer. Then imagine this with your knees and ankles.
7 It is quite likely that you will find your body taking some full breaths as the old body tensions release. Encourage this.
8 Visualise the legs moving up towards the ceiling, in the direction the knees are pointing.
9 Check through from head to toes. Is there any 'doing'? Is there another degree of letting go possible?
10 Open yourself to a sensation of spaciousness inside.

- Set aside a time each day (e.g. lunchtime, before dinner) to allow this deep letting go and opening out.
- The physical opening out will usually support a sense of emotional opening.

RELAXATION EXERCISE
Tension and surrender

A simple relaxation exercise to release deep tensions. Good to do before quiet work like meditation. It uses over-stressing to assist a deeper letting go.

- Lie on a carpeted floor, stretch out limbs, contract and expand your whole body a few times.
- Visualise yourself as a five-pointed star, with each limb and the head as a point.
- Begin tensing up body parts in this order:
  - right hand, right arm, hold for a moment, let go;
  - right foot, right leg, hold for a moment, let go;
  - left foot, left leg, hold for a moment, let go;
  - left hand, left arm, hold for a moment, let go;
  - face, trunk, hold for a moment, let go.
- Get a rhythm going: Tense! Tense! Hold! Relax! (In group work we use a drum beat to help establish the rhythm.)
- Go around the limbs about three times.
- Lie still. Feel yourself twinkling, pulsating like a star.

RELAXATION EXERCISE
Moving in slow motion

This simple exercise follows on from the tension and surrender exercise very well. It helps you become very conscious of your body. Move at a very, very slow speed to force consciousness to come into your limbs. Quiet flowing music will help.

- Lie on the floor with your limbs spread out a bit.
- Leaving your arms resting on the carpet, begin turning your wrists very, very slowly — so slowly that the movement is between the point of stillness and movement.
- Bring your whole attention to sense the movement, the subtle changes in the muscles as the movement continues.
- Leave your wrists after a while and explore your ankles. Allow your ankles to turn together or in opposite directions. It doesn't matter which direction; don't think about it, just feel the movement.
- Explore moving your neck in the same way.

- Work with an ankle and a wrist on opposite sides of the body; then change to the other ankle and opposite wrist.
- Now begin to include the neck. Don't think about it, lose yourself in the slow motion.
- Kneel up — let your upper torso turn through space — keep it slow! Add the wrists and neck, either altogether or one at a time.
- Stand — try moving every part so slowly, then allow your body to turn through space, let go of all control now, surrender to the flowing. Create your own Tai Chi.
- Rest, become still, stay attentive to the energy within you.

Meditation

There are many schools of meditation but in just this one chapter we do not have space to explore them all. Most meditations focus on one aspect of the process. For example, there are yoga schools that affect the inner energy through body postures. There are meditative methods that are designed to influence the heart and the emotions. Other schools prescribe mental exercises.

Some modern approaches try to graft on wonderful experiences or wonderful ways of thinking positively. This can give you brief periods of excitement but can subtly set up ego expectations and struggles with perceived failures. There is no substitute for your own will, intentions and perseverance. Meditation involves the paradox of the need for surrender and the need for willpower!

Some of the ancient practices of silent sitting — for hours — seem inappropriate to the modern person's lack of strong physical activity in daily life, or our deep tensions and agitation. We need to find a balance that is challenging without causing harm or more stress!

Why do we want to meditate anyway? Do we need to relieve stress? Are we tired of feeling that there is little meaning in what we do day after day? Do we want space for spiritual awareness? These questions are vital. Questions open you up. A state of questioning helps you delve deeper than the immediate needs of your ego.

Before trying to mediate ask yourself:

- Is there enough pleasure in the way I live my life?
- What does my ego want?
- What does my seeker part want?
- What are my essential aims?

Have you had enough of trying to fit into this world and trying to meet other people's expectations? Age brings many of us a sense that the old goals do not bring the fulfilment we had hoped for. We begin to realise that there is no new 'thing' that will make us feel better, that will make things complete. We may have tried to find a partner who would make us feel complete. This seems to work for a short time but eventually we return to the mystery of who we are and how we can experience life more deeply.

One of the pitfalls in learning meditation is that the role of the ego may intrude in a process which essentially must become ego-less. Any meditative activity — inner or outer — that remains directed by the ego will eventually lead to imbalance. The ego will have you strive for something already known. It usually aims at achievement, not surrender or discovery. Most commentators on meditation say that only through deep questioning and opening ourselves to the unknown within can new, healthy experiences and states evolve.

The journey inwards and the place of emotional release

The journey within goes through many different stages. Generally people in post-industrial societies have to do some emotional release work to expel the long-term effects of their social conditioning, which has focussed so well on outer achievement, but neglected just about all internal levels of consciousness.

These are some of my symbols for the stages you may go through before you can fully achieve a state of deep meditation:

The wild person within

Look inside yourself and it is quite possible you will find a wild person. Sometimes this wild person may be 'out of control';

crazed with endless chatter, a tortured body of contractions, and emotions so buried and held in that nothing in life seems relaxed or easy.

The bird in a cage

You may recognise that your tender side, your potential to be still and quiet, and your essence seem to be locked up. Your subtle potential is certainly alive, but it is restricted, enclosed, not free.

Army tanks

Perhaps you will find a battlefield inside. Vehicles of war confront each other, there are explosions, stand-offs, retreats, defeats and moments of victory. Almost all the parts of your personality seem to be at war. Confusion reigns although it may be well hidden from the world around you.

The tin man

The Tin Man from the Wizard of Oz is an apt symbol and description of how you may find your body when you become more conscious of it. When you take time to really connect with the sensation of your muscles you find armouring (see page 147). Your joints need a good oiling, and it seems as if — like the Tin Man — you have no heart.

The witch

You have spent most of your life pushing away your shadow but it is still there. When inner work begins and releases parts of your shadow personality you may feel like the old stereotype of a witch. She can lash out unexpectedly, even making you wonder if opening up your inner world was such a good idea.

An opening shell

When you have experienced emotional and physical release the image of the Tin Man gives way to the opening shell. As you take quiet time to be with yourself at a level deeper than thought, you may feel a natural desire to open, expand, and reveal the treasures within.

The snake

The snake or serpent has been a symbol for a strong flowing energy through many cultures and over many centuries. This lifeforce can sometimes be felt rippling through the body, sometimes up the spine, sometimes through every cell. Focussing your attention on this energy allows it to even out through the body and brings a feeling of bliss, groundedness and aliveness.

The pagoda, temple or cathedral

Depending on your cultural background you could use one of these as a symbol for something inside that now calls you to be still and quiet at times. The sacred space within — which has been symbolised externally by sacred architecture — becomes a more comfortable place to be. It remains a challenging place, but the challenge now is to remain attentive, present to a new space inside.

The hermit

Emotional release work has brought you many experiences of integration and peace. Now you look for new ways of directly entering the peaceful state. Deliberate periods of retreat from the world are needed to balance your expression in the outer world. Some of the best aspects of traditional religious life can now be integrated with your daily living: creating a routine for occasional withdrawal within yourself for replenishment.

The Buddha

Whatever your background and beliefs, the image of those very solid Buddha statues brings a feeling of earthy spirituality and centredness. In this stage your energies are recreated. When you find how to simply, yet actively, be with yourself, you will find more subtle, creative, focussed energy. This energy generates questions like: 'What should I do now? What am I here for? How can I serve?'

Meditation preparation questions

Take time to consider these questions, then write about them in your journal. Take plenty of time.

- What do you hope to achieve through meditation?
- What is your particular main obstacle to becoming quiet and still? Is it connected to agitated emotions, revolving thoughts or a restless body?
- What is the main thing you would like to change in yourself?
- What feels just right inside you? (e.g. 'I am a patient person')
- Is there an area of your body that seems more alive right now, where you can connect with your lifeforce?
- Do you ever experience a deep inner silence? If so what do you do in the silence?

Humans are between two worlds — material and spiritual. We embody the possibility of transformation: evolution of matter into spirit and the descent of spirit into manifestation. Our ultimate fulfilment depends on consciously supporting the evolution.

Since we are always being called by outer life, the main effort of meditation is focussed on hearing the call from the life inside us. This inner life needs our consciousness for its growth. On the highest level we serve the growth of spirit, of consciousness on the planet, and on our personal level we create conditions for a rich inner life of well-being.

Organised meditations are a preparation for daily life. Through meditation we not only come to truly see the outer world but as Krishnamurti says 'The knower becomes the known.'

There are three main stages in leading the meditative life.

1 Preparation, clearing, catharsis, releasing suppression.
1 Evoking the witness state — quiet work in complete surrender.
3 Meditation in action — bringing together all of ourselves, consciously, in daily life.

Meditation is ...

Meditation is inner adventure. It is being a witness with choiceless awareness. Through it we can become still and experience a poised, neutral state where we gradually learn to let go of tension, expectation, analysis and ego direction. Meditation includes a watchfulness of body sensation, emotional mood and emergence of higher or positive emotion. During meditation we can link up to our thinking state and watch the movement from revolving, automatic thoughts to quietness. We can sense the vibration of inner energy, the pulsing of lifeforce.

This delicate state — that most of us can only touch for a moment — includes a balance between action and non-action, remaining with the moment — now.

Meditation is not ...

In this context, meditation is not just any one specific technique. It is not simply mind activity — contemplation or introspection — thinking about things. It is not narrow concentration or limiting your range of awareness. It can be similar to prayer but it is not asking for something. It is not the same as active imagination or daydreaming or fantasy, although these may sometimes help us move towards a more quiet state. Meditation is not fulfilling to the ego.

Stages in quiet sitting meditation

These stages presume that the meditator has previously 'cleared' themselves through the emotional release methods described in this book.

1 Coming home — beginning to anchor awareness in the body.
2 Staying with an active effort to pay attention within.
3 Letting effort evolve into non-effort, becoming receptive to subtle sensations and energies within.
4 Breath relaxes and gains a nourishing quality.
5 Entering 'creative emptiness' — sometimes called the void — feeling new energy flow in while in this state.
6 Emergence of subtle positive feelings which are the result of your new harmony and new energy. People in this stage often say they feel bliss.

Walking meditation

Walking, which most of us do every day, can become a meditation. Some Buddhist monks work at it for years, and films of them in practice show the great subtlety of their steps. Their tradition obviously encourages inner focus, with the movements of the feet providing an anchor for the attention.

Most of us actually cling to the earth as we walk. Try this: go for a quick walk and observe — from the inside — how much tension there is in your ankles. Then try to walk and relax them at the same time.

Here are a few suggestions for how to turn walking — which you do every day — into an activity that will also further your inner exploration.

- Sometimes go for a walk just for the sake of inner observation, with no energy committed to where you are going and no need to arrive.
- Don't look at your feet but turn your attention to the movement of each foot. Feel the heel-sole-toe movement.
- Practise letting go at the ankles with each step.
- Try walking very slowly, feeling each nuance of change in the muscles. What is really involved in walking? Be in your legs.
- Go barefoot. Focus your interest to take in the textures and temperatures of the gravel, grass, cement, earth, road, etc.
- Walk with your inner awareness turned to your 'hara', or energy centre just below your navel. Let breath and energy flow right down into you.
- Tune into the rhythm of your steps, see if you can synchronise your breath with your steps in some way. Enjoy the rhythm.
- Use the rhythm of your walking to remind you to send your inner awareness into the limbs of your body. For example, four beats or steps while you focus on the sensation in one leg, then four for the next, then four for the arms, and so on.
- Try tuning your attention into two places at once! For example, make an inner connection with your feet as they touch the ground, and at the same time feel the breath coming in and out of your chest.

- After sitting still for fifteen to twenty minutes, focussing awareness within, try slow movements, then walking and keep the inner awareness.

All these ideas can provide you with ways to 'be at home' in yourself as you go shopping, walking to the post-box, bush-walking etc. When we are more at home we are able to take in the beauty around us, meet others more deeply, and find a new pleasure within.

SUPPORTING THE PRACTICE OF MEDITATION
Reviewing my inner practice

- What are the best conditions for your meditation practice? And what do you have to do to ensure you will not be disturbed?
- What are your best times for quietly turning within? Sunrise — when the world's energies naturally awaken? Sunset — when everything gradually becomes still (in nature anyway)?
- How could routine help? Is there a time each day? Is there a special place or spot that seems just right?
- How could ritual help? Ritual brings focus. Create your own small rituals to cross over the threshold from ordinary, everyday consciousness.
- Are there any special clothes that make you feel good, that would support your inner effort?
- Begin to recognise and list the main ways you fight with yourself (e.g. constant self-criticism, the division between inner focus and the need for entertainment).
- Become familiar with your 'yes' and your 'no' to changing internal gears and becoming still. For most of us it is the 'no' that wins. Ponder on the power of the 'no'. Affirm the reasons of the 'yes'.
- Truthfully list your expectations of meditation. What goodies does your ego want? Feel the difference between the wanting of the ego and the emerging patience of the real seeker within. Write about this.
- Do you recognise any preliminary work that you need to

do before becoming still and quiet, and feeling comfortable in your body are attractive aims?

- Who can you share your inner efforts with? Do you need to establish a new friendship in order to compare notes and encourage each other?

Preparation for meditation

Being quiet can bring calmness but it may only last a short while. We need to give ourselves many experiences of meditation; of making our body, heart and mind more willing.

Here are a few preparation activities to consider.

- Physical surrender and sequential relaxation.
- Movement, shaking and vibration to release and activate energy.
- Massage to help release muscular tension.
- Breath — using the rhythm of breath as an anchor for awareness, and also allowing the breath to flow all the way through the body.
- Sounding to release feelings and energy (e.g. shouting, singing, humming, sighing).
- Soft music to help you let go of the day and tune in to yourself.
- Hot baths to relax the body.
- Emotional release to expel inner distractions.
- Owning resistance — recognising that parts of your make-up do not want to work this way.
- Connecting with your body through quiet inner focus and systematic relaxation.
- Arranging longer periods of meditation in retreat settings.

You also need to recognise that meditation may lead you into both more stillness and the need to release more physically and emotionally.

Most of your initial work with meditation will be actively clearing your inner turmoil, letting the suppressions be thrown out. This is preparation for being truly still and awake. Almost every culture has dance rituals to allow this. Maybe we have to re-invent the wheel?

Buddhists aim to remove the five 'hindrances' — sensual passion, ill-will, sloth, worry and perplexity — from the mind before meditation. You may need to do the same, clearing negative emotions through cathartic release work. It is also important to allow harmonising of body and mind through structured movement (e.g. Tai Chi).

Dance will awaken body energy and use up excess nervous energy. Bioenergetic dance work allows us to mirror inner chaos with release methods, merging with chaos, expressing it totally so that harmony results. Along with dance, sounding and humming can be used to vibrate the inner energy system and recharge the brain.

Sounding opens the throat and encourages heart energy to flow more freely. Early Christians used repetitive prayers and songs for activating and harmonising the inner energy. Chanting is another useful preparation for centring before meditation, and there are a number of good tapes or CDs of chants that help to quieten and focus the inner world (for example, recordings by *On Wings of Song*).

Evoking the witness state

The witness state is a delicate balance of your attention where you watch what is happening within and without, without interference. It is a state that most of us can reach only after considerable practice and it is the ultimate aim of many meditation techniques. Phrases such as 'effortless effort' and 'being not doing' are used to describe it. Witnessing your thoughts, emotional reactions and body states will enable you to shift from identifying with them to finding a central earthing place inside you that is free. Your presence, your being, can then grow. Mostly we are simply lost — without a witness — in a sea of reactions to the world around us.

Here are some hints for beginning to work towards this state of observing without interfering, evoking the witness state, becoming free of ego control.

- Remind yourself why you are making the effort to meditate or, if you are not sure, keep this question alive.

- Acknowledge any resistance, recognise that parts of you do not want to be quiet or still and are more attracted to outer activity.
- Your posture for quiet sitting should ideally be balanced, naturally stable, with the least possible tension.
- It is usually best to close your eyes or gently fix them in one direction (e.g. on a candle).
- Breath should be soft, even and relaxed — never forced or contrived.
- Surrender is the ideal state to begin from. It is important to simply acknowledge if you do not feel surrender at the beginning. There will be a transition period when your habits of being active gradually die down.
- Nothing special is supposed to happen. There is no external guru to prescribe your experience. Most of us want instant results, whereas we need simply to practise. We do not know how long it will take to become still within.
- Any struggle proves that we do not yet know how to meditate. How can we transform the struggle and relax into a simple effort of focussed attention?
- Expectations take you away from the present. Some meditation techniques can inadvertently set up expectations. Meditation proves to us that we rarely live in or experience the present.
- Compassion for yourself is as essential as any discipline. Although you may find yourself lost in thoughts of the future and memories of the past, gently make the return to awareness now, again and again.
- Waste no energy on self-criticism.
- Once a sense of witnessing is attained, allow methods to drop away. There are progressive levels of witnessing; beginning with a body awareness experience, 'Me, aware of myself'. Gradually the 'me' fades and there is a new world of sensation, energy, truth, relaxation and centredness.

Dangers in unsupervised meditation

Meditation and prayer methods in old Western traditions utilised body energy and allowed for preparation of the mind. For example, the Greek Orthodox Church had many rituals that involved bowing, prostrating, sitting and standing. Most of us do not have this preparation.

Long strict sitting methods, such as Vipassana or ZaZen, should only be done under the direction of an experienced teacher, and usually not mixed with emotional release work. These techniques were designed for people leading a strenuous physical life. Unsupervised practice — where there is a clash of philosophy or an emphasis on control — can disturb our psyche.

Psychic phenomena such as the appearance of lights or auditory phenomena occasionally come into awareness, but they should not be given the focus. And most certainly not aimed for.

Identification with states and experiences touched in meditation is dangerous for balanced inner growth. Occasionally the ego will totally identify with some deep meditation experience. The ego is then said to be inflated. The meditator can then lose touch with groundedness.

Looking for results and pride in achievement are often associated with a rampant ego. Egos are usually trying to make up for some hurt or loss in childhood, and 'success' with meditation can be part of this. Without guidance a needy ego can grab on to meditation as another way to boost self-importance.

An ego-driven person will often be working only for personal gain, and from a strong self-will, not a surrendered place within. We should ask ourselves whether we seek something higher? Are we out for enhanced personal power? What do we do with the newly collected energy?

Impatience is a natural human trait. It will often surface during meditation practice. It has been said that 'forcible opening of a bud will not produce a blossom'. If you have been led to great expectations, some depression may follow. After all, our minds can be truly wild and our bodies chronically tense! Without support and peers to check out your reality, the sense of despair can sometimes be so strong that you abandon your attempts to learn meditation.

Mixing methods can be a complication for some. For example, sometimes emotional release work and quiet sitting do not go well together although many people find they do.

Different approaches may draw on different conceptual frameworks. It is best to be very clear about the background of the methods you are using and why you have chosen them. Experienced practitioners or teachers are invaluable here.

How can you tell if meditation is progressing?

Every day, at sunrise, while watching the reflection of its splendour, bring about a contact between your consciousness and the various unconscious parts of your general presence. Try to make this state last …

G. I. Gurdjieff from All and Everything

- You are more loving.
- Your inner silence becomes more accessible and deeper, or your ability to watch the chattering self without judgment or irritation increases.
- You establish a deeper connection to the energy in your body and feel more frequent sensations of its warmth, its vibrating, tingling or expansion.
- You have a stronger feeling of balance; a sense that you have located the true centre of gravity.
- You frequently feel 'at home', centred, present — the body begins to call you back home.
- Your inner reactions to others are not 'out of control'.
- Your senses become more vital; the trees seem greener, the air crisper, and the sounds you hear clearer and are more like music.
- You experience moments of waking up in daily life, of becoming present in action.
- All this brings you to great delight, a more stable view of life and a sense of meaning and purpose.

Karma yoga — meditation in action

Karma yoga is a way of inner attentiveness within the activities of daily life. The concept has been developed in the Hindu tradition as a way of preparing for our liberation from karma — repaying with consciousness generations of sleep. This way uses all parts of us, all centres. It can be further understood from the teachings of G. I. Gurdjieff, who introduced in this century a new synthesis of eastern approaches to consciousness evolution.

The idea of daily life as a yoga has the appeal of bringing together your times of focussed meditation and a way of learning more about yourself from the events and actions of each day. When the emotional, intellectual and physical parts of our psyche work together harmoniously we create an energy that can connect us to the Higher Self.

Meditation in action is a daily effort which can continue the transformation of energy begun in an early morning sitting. Karma yoga helps you maintain this precious energy. Normally we are like a sieve, filled each night with fresh lifeforce, awakening it powerfully in our active meditation, centring it in quiet work, and then leaking it out all through the day.

Sacred Psychology

Sacred Psychology is a term for the collected ancient and contemporary knowledge of our psyche in its normal state and its possible evolution. This knowledge, as it appears in a range of cultures and times, offers us the steps of development that can activate higher parts of ourselves and connect our psyche to what Jung called the collective unconscious. You can gain glimpses of this expanded realm through Transpersonal work, but you may find that prolonged contact may only be possible after considerable personal healing.

The path ahead, the path that takes us beyond the personal healing journey, calls for a very alive self-observation, a nonjudgmental watching for old habits. A new inner space is created by this continual inner watching, and a useful detachment to outer activities and inner reactions is generated. This self-observation has been cited by Krishnamurti and others as a starting point for the sacred journey.

After a good deal of healing work is complete you can develop the ongoing practice of awakening your energy and let it expand again and again. This will prepare the way for connection to the divine.

Becoming open to the spiritual level and letting it express

through you means clearing static, fine-tuning your personal self, and making progress at sensing the energy bodies — letting your awareness expand into them. Unlike your video-player or radio, you don't have a 'preset' button, where you can tune in and simply stay there. Your task is to be constantly tuning-in, finding the right frequency, focussing attention, until you pick up the messages.

For your part in supporting the manifestation of Spirit, you will need to develop will. It takes a force of will to stabilise attention within, to come into our natural functioning, to compensate for your old habits of scatteredness.

Perhaps you will know when you are on the right wavelength through a new sense of well-being. There will be an end to useless struggle and in its place an alert, subtle effort of attentiveness. This tuning-in will eventually allow the release of the blocks to your inner peace. After first revealing your inner turmoil and tension, it will support relaxation.

We all have the chance — through inner healing work — to connect deeply with and awaken the various parts of ourself, so that there will be harmony and a natural energy flow through the whole of us. This is the preparation, the fine-tuning of ourselves, necessary to co-operate with the expansion of Spirit.

The person who has found the way
Can pass on the gracious teachings to others;
Thus he aids himself and helps the others too.
To give is then the only thought
Remaining in his heart.

Milarepa, the Buddhist Poet-Saint
from *The Hundred Thousand Songs of Milarepa*
Vol. One Trans. Garma C. C. Chang (1989)

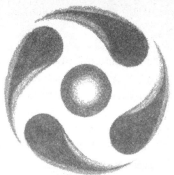

Forming Your Own Expedition
HEALING WORK WITH PARTNERS AND SUPPORT GROUPS

A relationship represents the greatest challenge for the individual, for it is only in relationship to others that unresolved problems still existing within the individual psyche are affected and activated.

Eva Pierrakos from *The Pathwork of Self-Transformation* (1990)

Healing work with your partner

Close personal relationships may be the most problematic area in your life. A close bond offers you the opportunity to carry your personal development into new levels of adventure and fulfilment. However, there seem to be fewer and fewer relationships that last well past the initial romance stage to actually become more life-giving and more loving. Disappointment in this area is widespread and deep. Many couples have given up and abandoned the adventure of sharing, self-revelation, mutual discovery and support.

This section of the book is designed to bring a deep re-evaluation of your beliefs and open you to new hope, to ways of bringing new life to relating. It contains many questions which should prompt and support your discovery of new answers.

There are several ERC concepts that relate to relationships which are explored here. The most important one is the idea that the unconscious has more real power — long term —

than the conscious mind. This is obvious when you consider how difficult it is to carry out your new resolves if unresolved unconscious emotions are influencing or blocking your conscious feelings. No matter how hard you try, you seem to make the same relationship mistakes over and over.

All strong relationships need maintenance. Popular magazines are full of advice on building up relationships but there is very little support for the deeper, soul-satisfying ways to strengthen relating. The truth is relationships require a constant commitment to relate, to open and to share. This rarely becomes automatic.

The bad news is that no amount or quality of maintenance will save a relationship if it is not based on adult love, respect and compatibility. The past will have left an imprint on how you relate. Your inner child may be leading you to establish unfulfilling and ultimately doomed relationships; the child keeps you hoping that soon — if you struggle hard enough — you will get it right. How long can this hope satisfy you?

A relationship begins with your relationship to yourself. How can you be present for another if you are not 'at home' in yourself? Because we are not normally brought up in our culture to be comfortable with our inner world it takes some regular effort to reach this stage.

Your soul, your inner world, wants you to recognise it, connect with it, not project it on to others. You may have searched 'out there' through partners for what you need to find in your journey of individuation. Relationships can begin to unravel with the recognition that the partner falls short of fulfilling all needs.

Sharing openly and honestly builds the bridge to the other. The art of building that bridge has to be rediscovered and practised over and over. Active listening (see page 109), being 'at home' to receive the other, helps build the bridge. Since we have all developed a layer of idealised self-image, this honest self-exposure can be very challenging and usually frequently needs outside help to begin.

Anything hidden is a barrier to a good relationship. The practice of keeping secrets builds a wall, and takes away the possibility of being known and accepted at a deep level. At the beginning of your healing journey you may feel the old need to keep some things secret, and yet have a longing to be known for all of your true self.

Initially, a problem in your relationship, or a blockage in creatively dealing with the problems, is usually in you, not 'out there'. Only when you have done your own personal clearing work can you clearly see what is out there in the other.

A flow of tenderness, love and sexuality can result from renewed connectedness or 'eros'. The word 'eros' here designates that special energy that creates empathy. It is an energy, or bond, that comes automatically at first as part of romance. It can be felt in groups gathered for healing work and will grow between a counsellor and client. It is like love; it connects you. This energy emerges when you are vulnerable and expose your inner self. Between couples it is a force that can be intentionally created by sharing the truth, sharing deep interests, sharing quiet times together. It is the force that renews the spark in marriage and long-term relationships.

The following exercises are for people who are ready to face themselves, for partners who wish to, or need to, understand more about their part in their relationship. The aim is to review your relationship and allow your inner world to guide you. The only risk in opening this topic is that you may find things you have been trying to ignore or avoid in yourself. The questions here could 'rock the boat' but the rewards include renewed and nourishing connections with yourself and others.

JOURNAL QUESTIONS
Reviewing my wish for a close relationship

Sit quietly and let each of the following questions reverberate inside. Write down your answer. Let your writing flow out without changing the words.

- What is your heart's desire in any relationship?
- What is your ideal of yourself as a partner?
- What does your inner child say about the risks of being honest and sharing openly?

- How ready are you to expose your deepest self — both the hidden beauty and the shadow?
- What is your main criticism of your partner?
- Is there anything similar you know you need to change in yourself, but have not done yet?
- What are the main triggers in your partner or close friends that 'set you off'?
- Is your main defence against being hurt one of withdrawal or explosion?
- What aspects of yourself do you fear to bring into a relationship?
- Is there a particular lack or 'hole' in your psyche that you want a partner to fill?
- Do you feel like sharing these answers with your partner?
- What have you uncovered that needs to be followed up either with your partner or a counsellor?
- Are there any tasks or new aims you need to set for yourself as a result of this exercise?

SELF-ASSESSMENT QUESTIONS
How do I relate?

You relate through ideas, knowledge, emotions, touch, sensations and energy links. Which of these ways do you use in relating? Write a line on each. Share your reflections as you go with your partner, or both write your answers at the same time, then share them.

1 Describe how you relate to yourself:
   Your unconscious _____ Your sexuality _____
   Your thoughts _____ Your lifeforce _____
   Your feeling _____ Your soul _____
   Your body _____
2 Describe how you relate to others:
   Family _____
   Colleagues _____
   Children _____
   Friends _____
3 Describe how you relate to special others:
   Your lover _____
   Your closest friend _____

4 Describe how you relate to the divine _____
   Your Higher Self _____
   God _____
   States of higher consciousness _____
5 Describe how you relate to nature _____
   Around your home _____
   In the bush _____
   Your favourite environment _____

The inner child in relationships

The healing journey often brings up memories of a poor relationship between your parents, and their inability to relate to you. You may have to go through feeling the pain of not having a good model. This pain was probably buried in infancy. After reliving these old memories and clearing your personal taboos on deep relating, you may find an active hunger to feel closer to people — to your friends in general and to a particular other in the deepest intimacy.

You begin to recognise previously unconscious, self-defeating and limiting ways of seeking relationships. You begin to recognise the moments of fulfilment in meeting another deeply, and to study the feelings and sensations of that wonderful state. You gradually become more expert at knowing if you are being used by your past to try to complete unfinished business of the hurt inner child.

Relationships can be used for the child's struggle to get what it did not get in the past. This is quite common. You often transfer the child's old ways of relating on to the present. For example, you may pretend to be present and attentive as the child did with parents. You may find that you remain 'unable' in some way in order to get help. Trying to please the other all the time is another child-motivated way of relating, or you may continue your childhood effort to be the peacemaker.

When the patterns of the past are activated you find a great need of the other, you no longer feel choice in relating and you find yourself more or less desperate for the other. If you believe you are empty you need the other to fill the hole. Or you may totally avoid relating and remain alone as a protection against feeling any past needs. Often you want to be given affection, approval, touch or entertainment. You almost want partners to be responsible for connecting you with the divine. As the child you frequently reacted to slights and neglect. Is this pattern clouding your perception now?

The hurt inner child has a long pattern in most of us of turning outwards for things. It did need love and comfort and warmth from without. It did need to be fed. But this pattern often makes you look to another for what can only come to an adult from within. Our culture and literature sees this turning outwards as normal. Advice columnists recommend that spouses focus on pleasing the other to maintain a marriage, as if the other is a victim needing rescue, needing pleasing, like a baby. This turning outwards is particularly clear when decisions have to be made, or there is a seeking of new direction in life. The need for the thrill of romance, the need for your sexuality to come from the other all show this old pattern. The habit of filling all your time with the other, never giving yourself quiet space to drop down into yourself, into your sensation, your feelings — all this grows out of the child's learnings.

When you are swamped by this neediness your natural adult desire and enjoyment of the other is eclipsed. Out of this neediness the inner child makes an issue out of momentary separations or the taking of personal space by the other whereas adult love brings a concern for the well-being of the other and the possibility of contentment whatever the external circumstances.

The bottom line is that you believe love comes from the outside, and so ignore the one place were you could actually find a regular supply of it — within yourself.

You may find that you put up with what the child believes you deserve. In this case abuse, unfaithfulness and neglect would seem natural and inevitable. You are 'on the look-out' for, and react to, perceived slights against you. The child's radar is alert for proof that the past is the truth.

Perhaps one of the most demeaning traits of the inner child's domination of you occurs when you exaggerate what is immature in your partner, even draw it out, in order to struggle with it, to try to change them. You find yourself playing games — reacting, sulking, demanding — in some old play that has the hopeless aim of extracting the love and care you needed from your parent(s). As a child you expected your parents to know what you needed. You can find that you don't ask for what you want now as an adult, still expecting it to be known.

Being overtaken by the inner child's reactions — or regressing — frequently follows a missed moment of true adult relating. These moments of relating often contain what you feel to be negative or unacceptable responses. For example, if an energy is aroused in you to challenge a statement made by your partner, or if you need to clarify something that he or she has said that seems hurtful, and the energy is not expressed the result may be a regression to the hurt child state.

If you don't share a feeling of hurt immediately, but dwell on it, brooding, withdrawal can result. We have all practised this withdrawal with our parents, this 'seeming to be', that is often a punishment to them. A sensitive partner will notice the changes, see how your body turns away, your voice drops, your muscles contract, your eyes glaze over. If they could see your thoughts they may see your plans of retreat and perhaps how you collect together all the reasons that prove separation is the only way to proceed!

A build up of energy and feelings also occurs as you notice the small daily differences in the way a partner does things. Every time you are reminded that your partner is not like the good side of Mum or Dad (or like God) or that they do things in a very different way from you, there is a reaction. If you don't take responsibility for yourself, or share truthfully or ask for the simple changes you want, the child in you comes to the fore — regression again!

One aspect of this child state is the belief that you can remain passive within yourself. For example, you may be drawn to a leader, to an entertainer, to a lover who can call up some energy in you. You may sit back in a deep inner armchair awaiting love, romance, connection to come to you. Of course, this belief is supported by old imprints from the time in the womb and the genuine need to receive everything from the outside from early infancy. However, the mature adult always has an interest in being active in a relationship and looks for new ways to give themselves. Passivity can govern much of your life until you challenge it.

Your inner child's desire for parental approval can be transferred on to your partner(s). Acting on an unconscious imprint you may hold back from being or living out your whole self. You may hide feelings from your partner that you learnt were unacceptable to your parents. This hiding of any aspect of yourself causes a distance and a closing of energy flow. Hiding interrupts deeper meeting that is a vital part of maturing relationships. You may also find that you withdraw from a partner emotionally whenever he/she exhibits a trait similar to something feared in the parent.

Accessing the childhood memories and influences that are locked up inside you, and recalling your childhood behaviour patterns, is a major step in preparing you to live and relate as a mature adult.

◆

Intimate relationships promote inner growth
A 48-year-old woman writes in her journal

The day my partner and I separated I had a dream which — when I worked with it — showed me a bonding pattern of the hurt inner child in relationships. The dream showed me that the pattern was to support the man so he wouldn't feel his negative feminine side. I would come in and prop him up. I'd be his life so he wouldn't feel the pain of his disconnection with his feminine. The dream showed the attachment which kept me from feeling the pain of the split from my own inner feminine. The hurt inner child took up a lot of space in my relationships. This space is now available for deeper relating and creativity.

A DRAWING EXERCISE
Turning within for self-discovery

This exercise can be done purely for your own self-knowledge and practice. It is also good to do this work at the same time as your partner so that your discoveries can be shared. Every time you share more of what is inside it helps create a deeper bond.

Have some good quality crayons and large drawing book or paper ready.

- Draw a large outline of your body.
- Find out what is going on inside you. Relax totally. I suggest that you lie down on cushions or thick carpet. Become still. Tune in to your body. Notice:
  - physical sensations
  - feelings
  - energies.
- Express what you found on the body outline. Choose colours, lines and shapes carefully for each of the three experiences.
- Date the drawing, and repeat this exercise at least once a week for a while.
- If your partner is there share your drawing with them.
- At some future time take out your body outline drawings and notice what has changed and what seems the same.

Relationship-building exercises for willing partners

All these suggestions are designed to break through barriers that may have grown between partners. In most cases, the suggestions will bring some resistance. Acknowledge this and then proceed. Dare to hope for new aliveness, reconnection and renewed closeness!

Exercise 1 — Active listening

This is a way of listening to each other without interrupting, answering, justifying or commenting. You listen to the feelings in what is being said, not just the story.

- First tune into yourself, then become like a barometer, simply listen and register.
- Focus on emotional content not just rational content.
- Each person takes a turn at telling an important episode in the story of their life. The partner listens, then shares what they heard of your feelings and energy underneath the words.

Exercise 2 — A bonding exercise for couples

Sharing your thoughts, feelings, experiences, hopes and dreams enlivens your bonding. The assumption here is that both partners do want to be closer. Often these exercises can activate your old defences and bring to the fore parts of yourself that would like to ridicule inner work and anything that makes you vulnerable. It will help if you share your worries openly. A sense of ritual in setting the space for this exercise will reinforce what you are hoping to do and the importance of finding a way forward individually and together. Remember that real growth in relationship is a rare thing. If you have a partner who is willing to go through this exercise, you already have a lot!

Organise some quiet time when you will not be interrupted — at least an hour and a half. (If you cannot do that, skip this exercise and examine your lifestyle!)

- Take the phone off the hook.
- Have a box of tissues handy.
- Sit facing each other.
- Close your eyes and take a few minutes to tune in to yourself first.
- Take six slow, full breaths and relax them out.
- One partner will share first. The other partner reads out the questions below, one at a time. This partner may not interrupt, comment, add, argue, respond or defend.
- Before you respond to the questions share what is happening inside you now. Share any resistance to doing this exercise together, any fears.

Bonding questions

- What did you learn about relationships from your parents?
- What do you know about your own self-love and self-hate?
- Outline what have been the high points and the low points in this present relationship.
- Share the deepest longing in your heart.
- Share any image you have of how the relationship could grow.
- Is there a fear about letting the relationship go deeper?
- What is really important now?

- When both of you have responded, lie down and tune in again.
- Take some full breaths.

- Contact:
  - your feelings
  - your energy
  - what is happening in your body
  - any fantasies that are alive in you now.
- Sit up and share what is going on inside you now.
- Be aware of what your energy is wanting now. Solitude? A brisk walk? Making love? A celebration? Can you share that?

Exercise 3 —Reading and studying together

Set aside some time to discuss books about relationships or, better still, read something together. There are some excellent texts that can be read together and discussed as a first stimulus to opening to more in your relationship.

Recommended books:

Robert Johnson, *The Psychology of Romantic Love*, Arkana, Britain, 1987

Eva Pierrakos, *The Pathwork of Self-Transformation*, (chapters on the inner child and relationship), Bantam, USA, 1990

Eva Pierrakos & Judith Saly, *Creating Union*, Pathwork Press, USA, 1993

Exercise 4 —The ideal and the actual

Take turns talking and listening:

1 List all your ideals of how you should be as a partner. Tell your partner about yourself and your idealised self-image as partner/lover.
2 List all the characteristics of your ideal partner/lover. Really let yourself exaggerate — is this desire for such absolute perfection humorous?

Exercise 5 —Wordless exchanges

Line and Colour

- Have some large paper and good crayons ready.
- Express your inner state with line and colour at the top of the page.

-   Your partner draws a response on the same piece of paper.
-   You respond to their response by drawing again.
-   Continue in this way until you get to the bottom of the page.
-   Your partner now begins at the top of the next page, and you respond.
- Now express your feelings and attitudes together in a mandala.

Touch

- Take turns using touch only to communicate.
    -   Sit opposite your partner.
    -   Your eyes are closed.
    -   Think of something definite you want to convey and say it with touch.
    -   Your partner says what they think you meant.
    -   Repeat until the communication is clear.
    -   Change roles.

Exercise 6 — Letting go of old bonds

1 Talk about the major bonds or relationships you have had in the past that still haunt you, or with which you compare your present relationship (e.g. previous marriages).
2 Talk about the high points and the low points in those past relationships. Try not to hide anything. Be prepared to feel any emotions that may still exist in you. For example, is there still some grieving to be done, or anger/fear to be released?
3 Watch for any reactions such as jealousy, comparison or inferiority in yourself or your partner. Discuss these frankly.

Transforming relationship difficulties

This section explores some aspects of transforming relationship difficulties into growth-promoting challenges. The old bonds of marriage used to force this to happen to some extent, but today the usual response to difficulties is to turn away, or walk away, blaming the other.

There is a deep need in the human psyche for experiences of transformation. Over your lifetime, you may feel impossible hate and distance turning again into love and closeness; or passive acceptance that you cannot have what you want may become the excitement of actively taking hold of all possibilities.

The following questions are designed to activate thoughts, memories and emotions. They may make you feel uncomfortable. They may stir up some new insights. They will give you a basis for confronting relationship problems as a positive exploration. Use them as a checklist for deepening communication with your partner and/or as a way to encourage your personal reflection or journal writing time.

Pondering, journalling and sharing questions

Your self-exploration

- Is it more important to concentrate on yourself or your partner?
- Do you have a commitment to your own inner journey?
- Do you think it is selfish to devote time to understanding yourself?

Reactions

- What are the main hurts in your life now?
- Is rejection and fear of rejection a deciding factor in what you do or do not say to your partner?
- Do you recognise the triggers that set off your strongest reactions?
- What do you do with your anger?
- Do you have any safe outlets for your anger?
- Are you able to find the hurt underneath reactions of anger?
- Are you ready to expose your vulnerable side to your partner?

Projections

- Can you find some of the positive qualities you see in your partner in yourself?

- Can you find some of the negative qualities you see in your partner in yourself?
- Are these qualities more or less acceptable in yourself?

Lack of energy between partners

- What has been depressed inside you? Think back over the last few days or weeks. Are there any feelings or statements that you may have pushed out of sight.
- Is there something you have kept hidden from your partner?
- Have you forgotten to share your inner world recently?

Fear of depth in relationship

- Is there anything you fear in your partner?
- Is there anything you fear your partner finding out about you?
- Are you aware of any fear of powerful sex?
- Is there some fear of revealing yourself emotionally?
- Have you been hiding yourself spiritually?

Wholeness versus perfection

- Have you ever found yourself thinking 'unless it is perfect it is no good'?
- Who is your model of a perfect partner?
- Do you have daydreams of some future time when things will be better or perfect?
- Is there a strain from trying to be, or get things, right?
- What does 'wholeness' mean to you in a relationship?

Male/female differences

- Men: Are you criticised for being too rational?
- Women: Are you criticised for being too emotional?
- Do you wish your partner had more active or receptive energy?
- Do your arguments become a clash of rational versus emotional viewpoints?
- Do you wish your partner thought more like you?
- Do you agree or clash on the differences in how you do the same task?

A ROLE-PLAY EXERCISE
Becoming my partner

- Take a moment to simply become your partner:
  - Stand or sit exactly like your partner.
  - Hold your body as they do.
  - What is their most typical facial expression? Make it.
  - Mimic their hand gestures.
  - What are the most common phrases they say? Say them in their voice.
- As you are playing around with this, feel inside and try to discover whether there are similarities with yourself. What are the main differences?
- You are, of course, playing your version of them, but how does it feel to be in their shoes? What do you think is their inner attitude towards themselves?
- How do you feel about them now in the light of these insights?

Understanding your way of relating

You can support further self-exploration as you go about the daily business of relating. Work with your journal, record your observations on how you relate to friends and a special other. Couples can use the following guidelines as a basis for discussion, opening to a more detailed sharing of the high points and dissatisfactions in your present level of relating.

The ideal you

An idealised self-image of yourself as a partner may stop you seeing how you truly are as a partner. Carrying a firmly-held ideal may make you an active critic of the actual you. Do you put yourself down all the time? Certainly a fixed ideal will hinder knowing the shadow side of yourself in relationship. If a relationship feels stuck or dead you can be sure that much of the life is held in the shadow, along with the aspects of yourself that do not match your idealised self-image. Always trying to live up to your idealised image (or another's ideal) is exhausting and phony. It is certainly no basis for a long-lasting relationship.

Be willing

Keeping love alive depends on your willingness to expose more of yourself, to contact and reveal your never-ending depths. How ready are you for emotional, physical and spiritual intimacy?

Active listening

In active listening you hear the feelings and energy 'state' underneath what the other is saying, not just the meaning of the words. You listen to the whole person, including their body language. You make an effort to stay open to hear the other, not just your own inner voices. It needs to be practised regularly to prepare you for difficult times when you are in reaction to the other. Practising quiet centring of yourself is extremely helpful here.

Mirroring

After listening actively, you can feed back the whole message you have heard from the other person. At the same time you need to avoid being caught in the rational meaning of the words. It does not matter if you are correct, the fact that you have listened carefully will help the other also listen more carefully to the whole of themselves. This will create a greater connection than rushing in with your point of view.

Occasionally, when you feel very attuned to the other person, you may be noticing their gestures, postures and subtle facial expressions. Whether or not you have some clue about what all this means, you can draw their attention to what is happening. This makes it possible to examine what may also be happening on an unconscious level, beyond the rational arguments or stories. Our bodies don't lie. This sense of watching should also be applied to yourself.

Needs

What are the gaps or holes in you that your partner fills? Do you feel less when you are apart? Is there a quality or characteristic that you need from them? When you believe 'I need' something the inner child has not been heard/seen/felt, but is acting through you, through your relating. Adults do desire and want things, but an energy of need comes from unfulfilled past needs of the child.

The unconscious hurt inner child

What did you learn about relationships as a child? What were you longing for in the way your parents related to each other? What is your inner child's intention for your relationship? Is it positive or negative, helpful or destructive?

What did you learn, through the experiences of your childhood, about the risks of being honest, sharing openly?

Reactions

What are your key powerful emotional states that are triggered by something your partner says or does? You usually say your partner causes your reaction, but it is your reaction. When you are in a state of reaction your own unconscious material is in the way of relating directly and cleanly.

Responses

You respond when you are in an adult space, relating to another, here and now, with no shades of the past intruding. From where in yourself do you know the difference between response and reaction?

Withdrawal

This indicates that a reaction has set in. You may seem to be present, but are really closed emotionally, and usually contracted in your body. In this state no real contact is possible. It usually means that you want to keep safe from feeling some old emotional pain that has been triggered.

Dumping

Emotional explosion and dumping, blaming the other for your feelings, is the opposite to withdrawal. Neither reaction is helpful in building your relationship; both must be recognised and worked with if they are your patterns of self-defence. Which way do your reactions tend to take you — implosion or explosion? What are the effects of telling your partner the negative feelings? Is it really productive?

Projection

Something unknown in you wants to emerge, but you are out of contact with it. You think you begin to see it in the other person. There may be some of this feeling or quality in the other, but you are seeing or fearing or wanting what is really in you. In this state you do not really see the other. This takes place unconsciously.

- What emotions/qualities do you disapprove of in the other?
- What emotions or qualities do you most fear in the other?
- What do you most admire in the other?
- Are any of these really in you?

Criticism

When you notice deep criticism of partners or friends you need to ask yourself:

- 'Is there something I need to do, but am not doing?'
- 'Am I wishing the other will do it for me or change in some way so that I don't have to?'
- 'What new steps do I have to take to renew relationship with myself and with the other?'

Anger

Your anger is often a cover for emotional pain. It is a reaction to being hurt. Anger insulates you from hurts, both past and present. It raises your defences and energy. You often feel alive and strong when angry. Can you risk being vulnerable and finding the sadness under the anger?

Resentment

This familiar mood killer follows a missed moment — a time when you did not express feelings or words in an adult way. You may use the other person to stop you being true, and blame them for it. Resentment leaks out like poisonous gas. It is held in the body and affects you. It is saved up and can be let out at times when the other is more vulnerable. Release comes from tracing back through time, finding the missed moment and recognising what you have done.

These ideas can form a basis for discussion and exploration together of new ways of relating. They can support your self-responsibility. It is not advisable that you analyse everything you do and say. The aim is to become more conscious of your interactions so that you can grow more positive together and become more spontaneous.

Summary — steps towards a more fulfilling relationship

- Know what you are feeling. Become used to connecting with yourself, practise developing the relationship with yourself.
- Make a commitment to this self-knowing and self-connecting. Let it become an ongoing practice, a journey. This commitment will bring life and freedom and clarity to your outer relationships.
- The development of relationships depends on continual discovery of each other. This begins with:
  - self-discovery
  - sharing what you discover
  - listening to the other's discoveries.
- The energy of love, of sex and of sharing deep friendship (eros) is different. In the mature, intimate relationship all three grow together, bringing more life. Begin to recognise these three energies.
- Most problems of distance, withdrawal, reaction, anger and irritation with partners have their beginnings in the hurt inner child. Relating more deeply will bring up the old feelings that you had as a child about your family, especially your parents. Be ready to deal with these and possibly seek experienced help.

  Discover your hurt inner child's script for relating to others. Begin to catalogue its main beliefs and behaviours, then you can go through feeling what the child could not. In so doing you can work free, and continually separate from its way of behaving. You can then relate as yourself, with maturity.
- You usually begin a relationship with preconceived ideas. You presume to know the other and/or unconsciously expect to be known and understood. Frequent and regular communication is essential to bring connection and

expansion to a relationship. Practise being direct and clear and honest. This requires you to know yourself first, and take the risk of being rejected.

- Begin to discover any previously unconscious idealised self-images you hold for yourself. There will be tension in the relationship if either of you is struggling to maintain an image of yourself.
- Begin to discover any ideals you hold of how a partner should be. Do you measure your partner against your ideals? These images (often resulting from the inner child's past needs) block you really meeting your partner.

All relationships have a natural movement of expansion and contraction, opening and closing and opening again. You should frequently take the risk of dropping your defences. Most anger, most distance, most arguments are efforts to keep our defences intact, to stay closed and 'strong'. Learn to simply drop under these defences and feel the vulnerability, the fear, the hurt that may be in you. This will allow the barriers around your heart to fall away, and it usually helps the other person to soften and open again too.

◆

Relationship problems
A 50-year-old man writes in his journal

I can't really be all of my real self around her. I realise that I choose to pay attention to her all the time, rather than giving time to connect with my inner self. I suspect my inner self feels neglected, even jealous of her. I want the joy within to be reflected in our outer life together, but I have been focussed on getting all my joy from interaction with her. My spiritual practice, my meditation has been abandoned.

When I relaxed, tuned in and took some deep breaths, I found that my inner self wanted to speak out strongly. It said:

'You have got to come back to me! Get a hold of yourself. You won't get what you want through humans. All joy, pleasure, fulfilment, peace and creativity come from ME. Enjoy your partner if you want to, but come back to me. Do not let the child's old longing for outer bliss and connection blind you to me. Get a hold of your child!'

The hurt inner child wanted to respond:
'I am ready to abandon everything for comfort, love, touch from the outside. My need is the greatest thing in you!'

After my emotional release work I decided to focus on these steps:

- To ritualise my morning meditation time and to make known my need for space and quiet.
- At the end of the day, to take time for me. Go to the other room to tune-in or dance and prepare to go to bed and connect with her in a more aware state.
- Deal with all my little reactions around the house as they arise, instead of storing them up so that they need to explode.

Support groups

While the rewards of the healing journey are countless, coping with the highs and lows along the way is often tough. Because we all have contradictory natures and periods of inconsistency seeing the way ahead can be really difficult at times.

It is very helpful to find some outside acceptance until you really accept the full range of what is within. You need the love and support of others until you grow enough self-love.

Many people benefit from a supportive healing group. In a group you can explore your inner work and its links to daily life. Groups can encourage you to be undefended, to drop your old need to keep ego barriers in place.

A bond will gradually develop and deepen within any group of people interested in the healing journey. Such a bond will help you discover a reverence for all life. Creating this bond takes long work, commitment, a focus on aims, and the risk of giving generously without expectation.

These groups are almost like scientific laboratories. We are the experiments. We study and work with our reactions, interactions, repulsions and affections. Noting these, and going forward together, lights a fire, like the alchemist's fire that melts all the elements together, and creates new materials, new states. Since ERC brings the possibility of continual new discoveries, these groups can become alive research groups, the meeting places for sharing new ideas, for exploring new methods, for understanding the functioning of the human psyche more clearly.

A support group is not simply for hand-holding. It should challenge you by contradicting old dysfunctional imprints of relating which may have been learned in your early years. They help map new fulfilling ways to live — calling up and drawing out the gifts of each member. These groups do not replace the need to find fulfilment in outer life. They are not social clubs in the old sense. In fact, in some cases, group members may appear to be the last people on earth who would plan to spend leisure time together. Your commitment to keep the journey alive is the bond that propels you past your first impressions and into facing your likes and dislikes as messages from your own psyche about yourself.

Any group can seek help from people who have journeyed longer. Groups that have been together for a while can create programmes for self-help and for community support. You should feel great support for your journey of growth and healing from being part of an inner work group. In the life of such a group there will be periods when professional guidance is essential, both for the group dynamics and for focussing on issues of deeper growth.

The question of leadership in a group can be a tricky one because some of us prefer to be followers and some want to be leaders. However, in a healing group I suggest that every member would strive to lead themselves. We may question the motives of someone who needs to have a group to follow him or her, and question our motives if we find that we are constantly feeling in need of someone to follow.

A group may need to have a limited life and a clearly defined (even if changing) aim. It is important that the group is not supportive in the sense of creating dependence. Group work is really preparation for your interaction, survival and real growth in the outer world. But I have also found that even the most accomplished professionals will choose to have a peer group to support and review their own inner direction.

You need only have four or five people to form a group. Why don't you mention the idea to friends or acquaintances at yoga classes, tennis club, or parent group? Sometimes a few couples gather to exchange their ideas and observations, or to read through a workbook to stimulate ideas. This book is designed to assist such groups and you could collectively work through the exercises and share your discoveries. It is ideal to include someone experienced in group work and personal journeying. The contacts at the back of this book could be of help here.

Outline — working with a group

Here are a few points to consider as you begin working with others:

- Your group is a research group rather than only a support group.
- It is necessary to create trust before people open up and deep sharing is possible. However, trust comes from shared healing work and taking the risk of self-exposure.
- Begin group work with a tuning-in and inner focus time.
- Explore active listening. Begin really listening to each other. Listen to the feelings carried in the voice not just the meaning of the words.
- Mirror back feelings, accept feelings, acknowledge them, rather than always trying to do something about them.
- Watch how you project your own feelings and expectations on to others.
- Begin to recognise emotional triggers. What, in others, sets your reactions off? Reactions to each other are inevitable. They will be helpful for your self-discovery, but only if they are acknowledged as being internal, about you, not the trigger.
- Listen to your own inner child. Is it demanding something?
- Become more comfortable in sharing your inner emotional state; practise sincerity by acknowledging what you are feeling.
- Form clear guidelines together about feedback. Each member should feel safe to share their inner world without comment from others, or to request feedback when they feel ready.
- Consider sharing massage as a way of letting the body feel direct support. It could be simply shoulders, feet or face and scalp.
- Support each other in taking time for deep relaxation. Although this idea is given lip service in our society, each of

us usually feels guilty if we take time to relax. Members could take turns at preparing and presenting a relaxation exercise (see pages 83 to 86).

- In deciding on new approaches and new directions, ask the question 'How will this support self-responsibility?'
- Make sure you take some time to refocus your awareness on yourself during group work. Don't get trapped into offering support all the time, or covering your own needs by constantly giving.

Beginning to meet on a deeper level

Some of the ideas in this section suggest a very high level of self-responsibility for members of a support group. Obviously it may take time for this to develop. Certainly a trained and experienced group facilitator could guide you towards enhanced awareness over time. Also these ideas become more relevant as you come up against the challenges of group interaction as well as the experience of good group support.

If possible, before talking with others about healing work, or before a group meeting, take time to come home to yourself. Taking time to centre yourself creates a better starting place for relating to others.

In a support group it is not ideal to sit on an issue or a problem that is alive for you. This holding back can regress inner healing work particularly if the issue is connected with the group or someone in it. Always share what is happening for you; find the right moment to express any reactions or reservations or strong excited energies. Once you embark on the journey it is vital that you avoid adding to the internal load of repressed issues and feelings.

If you are aware of it, always voice any resistance to being vulnerable or to sharing your inner world with the group. Share your worries or concerns because they are a force, and resistance is a force. You need to integrate that force, not alienate it and make it stronger. Express resistance. Once resistance becomes conscious and is shared it seems to be diminished. And then, of course, it won't hide in the background and spoil things, becoming the strong silent 'no' to our conscious 'yes'.

When you are not in contact with your feelings they are sometimes projected on to others. This is an unconscious mechanism. What is really inside you seems to be coming to you from the outside. For instance, if you feel that someone is reacting to you, or the group is reacting in some way towards you, then you need to ask if it is true. Is it really out there, or a feeling inside you?

If I am informed by what I see in another, if I simply register information, then my observation is probably valid. If I am affected, if I am in reaction, agitated, upset or outraged, what I thought was an observation may be a projection. Reactions are a good indicator for areas in your personality that need some reflection and perhaps some emotional release work. On the healing journey your task is to own your reactions. If you react to something the source of upset is inside you. Normally when you react you try to change the person who triggered the reaction. For the journey it is important to study what is going on inside you.

Reactions are a major source of self-study material. How does your body react? What trains of thought are initiated? 'Over-the-top' reactions can be used in emotional release processing (see page 158) to release more of the inner child hurts and to reclaim your adult self.

Each of us can be a mirror for others. Other people may actually see some of what is inside us, but frequently they see reflections of themselves. If I am really annoyed by something a group member says or does I need to look within myself and see if it is there also. For example, if I am very upset that someone is greedily taking all the time in the group, I may have to examine my own desire to be listened to. Normally we arrange our lives to have friends who will not mirror an aspect of ourselves that we would prefer not to accept.

Individuals are responsible for their own healing journey — not the group, a facilitator, support people (or even authors). The purpose of group work is to learn more about yourself, so try to maintain an attitude of gladness for all situations that give you a learning opportunity.

It is good to ask for support when some difficult issues or insights emerge in your journey. For example, you may suddenly realise that you have been carrying a deep resentment towards a sibling, and feel shame about this. But most of us operate from an unconscious belief that there is no support — usually it is the inner child who learnt that. Perhaps you are used to having no support and suffering in silence and alone? Don't overlook the fact that there are others around who are willing to support you if approached. You may need to break an old habit and form a new positive one.

Groups must clearly affirm that nothing personal from any member's journey will be shared outside the group. This is absolutely essential and, if you know a breach of confidentiality has occurred, it should be discussed immediately. This confidentiality is part of the basic conditions that make a group a safe place. Great psychic damage, as well as social damage, comes from divulging group content. This affects both the person who is talked about and the person who gossips. If you do discover a tendency in yourself to break confidentiality, to gossip, it can lead you to a deeper self-investigation.

Feeling tired during or after group work can be an interesting indicator. Ask yourself, and maybe check with the group, whether you are physically tired, or are you holding down feelings or issues? Repressing feelings and reactions is exhausting! When newly emerging unconscious material is about to break free your old defences must work much harder and it takes up more of your energy to preserve the status quo.

Holding down anger or rage uses your reserves of energy. Holding excitement and joy out of sight — as many of us have learned to do — is also exhausting. When you realise how you have misdirected your energy you can release it and experience a new aliveness.

Anxiety in a meeting is usually constricted excitement. Anxiety often emerges in group work. Tune in to it, then let the energy be free. You may need to stand up and stretch and shake your body or dance. Let energy flow again and then tune in: is it really joy, pleasure, sexuality, lifeforce?

Paying attention to other group members tests your compassion. How long do you remain interested in another's story? What happens in your heart? What does your inner child begin to say when someone else is getting all the attention? How can you stay connected and alive within while attending to another?

Give yourself, and each other, permission to be quiet in a group. It is not always necessary for your attention to be directed outwards. Socially that is what we are taught to do, but in a healing group we are more interested in creating an atmosphere of inner focus. Get into the habit of balancing your sharing and chatting with a little quiet space to reconnect within.

The value of sharing and the art of listening

Sharing your life and inner world experiences will clarify your thoughts and feelings. Listening to other people's stories also encourages you to reflect on your own.

Be very clear on the group dynamics. Who is sharing? Who is listening? Is there a designated facilitator or chairperson? How are the quieter members of the group supported to take all the time they need?

The person sharing does not have to have all the words and understanding ready and clear before starting. Many of us think we have to be clear first. The sharing is a clarifying process and hopefully your insights will change and deepen as the sharing progresses.

Drawings and mandalas can be a good starting point for anyone who does not feel confident verbally or who is still unclear about what they want to share.

Listeners should continually come back to a focus on their own heart area, and listen from there. The listener's attention is divided between the speaker and themselves. This supports objectivity, clarity, and a deeper level of caring. This work to 'be at home' will also support the listener to not identify totally with the sharer and thereby lose contact with themselves.

Make an effort not to analyse or tell another group member what their experience means. Even though it may be exciting, try not to intrude your interpretation of another's experience. This robs the speaker of self-discovery and can lead in a direction that is not truly theirs. A supportive group or group facilitator should never offer their opinions or negate what is being said. Your aim should be to draw out the speaker and, perhaps, help them examine what they are saying. Any interaction should lead towards self-discovery.

Sometimes it can be helpful to support the person sharing to move from generalities to specifics, if she/he appears ready. Staying general in a sharing situation is a way of keeping emotional distance. For example, a person may say 'Someone should really have taken care of me when I was little!' Do they mean mother or father? Or someone may say 'People should give credit where it is due!' Do they really mean 'My boss should tell me my work is good'.

Sharing in a group can involve some risk-taking. Group discussion is often the first test of a new truth or discovery and can be more challenging than individual revelation with one friend or counsellor. For example, a group member may talk about 'being a doormat'. They may be explaining it and find themselves interrupted. They may have to summon the courage to go against their old imprint — in which the interruption would seem normal and okay — and speak up and reclaim the space to continue.

A group is able to support members to express, formulate and record new truths and new intentions. Writing a summary of the discussion can be helpful. Summarising forms a ritual that brings a sense of order and ownership. A succinct summary of insights and truths makes them easier to remember.

An experienced group facilitator will offer help that links up the inner work experience to life now. The speaker may be invited to consider adult steps, such as new directions for career or relationships, or further specific integration activities.

◆

Beginning to work with a healing group
A 34-year-old man writes in his journal

I felt I was separate from the group. I could see my mind revolving all the time. I saw that I ridicule others, silently inside myself. My eyes were searching around the circle and I see faults in them all the time. I ridicule sentimentality and lack of presence — especially when they do emotional release work in the middle. This was happening strongly inside me. Suddenly I realised that this is how my mother always was towards me!! What was done to me — I now do! I felt much more alive when I accepted this. This ridicule is part of my shadow side.

Then I asked myself, 'Well, what are you looking for in the others?' The answer was 'a sense of being true, sincerity, at homeness.' I realised that I was wanting this to come to me, through the group, from the outside. I was looking OUT not IN for it. This is how I was as a child. With these realisations I felt my interest and awareness return to me. My chest felt more open, my breath seemed to relax and a great feeling of well-being came over me. I could feel the energy and support of the group. My previous decision never to do any release work in the middle of the group had been made by my hurt inner child! Will I be brave enough to make a new decision?

A few ways to begin first meetings

Groups need to be clear about leadership right from the start. Is there a professional facilitator? Are they all equally experienced to lead? Will there be a roster for being the leader? Often support groups have a roster of those who will take the lead role and design some starting points, choose some introductory centring or inner focus exercises.

Since the purpose of the group is different from the usual social interaction, it is usually helpful to have a structure to the meeting that formalises or ritualises the cross-over from social interaction to inner world focus. This ritual crossing of the threshold can simply be a few minutes of silent meditation, pondering of aims and needs, journal writing, relaxation, or drawing time.

It is always a good idea for members to have personal journals and pens at the ready, as well as drawing books and crayons. Some group members may be very articulate, or they may write very clearly, or they may prefer to express themselves with pictures. All these methods are helpful in exploring the inner world and can be used so that all members find a way of opening up that helps them most.

Meetings may begin with a facilitator or chairperson presenting some inner focus work. This may include the following six steps:

- An overview of the exercise.
- Silent or quiet focus on the inner world.
- Time for guided reflection or sensing what is inside.
- Time for expressing what is found (e.g. drawing, writing).

- Time to share and listen to others (either one-to-one or with the whole group).
- Feedback from the group on the exercise.

Here are a few exercises to begin first meetings. The instructions would be presented by the leader or professional facilitator.

1 Inner focus — finding a deep wish for growth

- Draw a large circle in a book or on paper.
- Come home into yourself; let your eyes close, sense your energy.
- Take a breath into the centre of your body.
- Focus awareness on the heart area.
- Consider the question, 'What is my inner longing now?' Wait, and let your longing surface.
- Draw a mandala of now.
- Write your responses to the question in your journal.
- Share your experience.

2 Body focus

- Have a body outline drawing and crayons ready.
- Come home into yourself.
- Direct your awareness through your body from head to toes.
- Check what is in each part of your body; feelings, sensations, pains, tensions, high energy spots.
- Express your observations on the body outline drawing with line and colour.
- Share your discoveries with others.

3 Sharing of backgrounds

- Arrange two concentric circles of cushions or chairs in pairs. The number of cushions/chairs coincides with the number in the group.
- Choose a partner and sit opposite each other. Introduce yourselves if you have not met before.
- Read through the list of questions (see below).
- Before you discuss each question you must become still, close your eyes, take a deep full breath and feel what is going on inside.

- When you have had a moment of inner contact the group leader will read out a question. Leave your eyes closed and wait and see what presents itself in your mind. Ponder the question for a moment. When both of you are ready to talk open your eyes and share your thoughts.
- After a few minutes those sitting in the outer (or the inner) circle stand and move on to the next cushion/chair on their right.
- Vary the number of questions to suit the time available and the interest level. If there is time you can choose a partner to meet with from your own circle as well.

Sample questions

- What things irritate you most in your life now?
- What is your strongest or best quality?
- How many brothers and sisters do you have? Where do you come in the family? How do you feel about that?
- What things make you sad at the moment? What things make you most happy?
- Is there anyone in your life you are afraid of?
- How do you feel about being in this group right now?

4 Using sandplay symbols

- Draw a large circle in a book or on paper.
- Visualise or imagine your life at the following ages. Imagine the setting and if you can remember the feelings that went with these ages. This may include what you were told about the early years, what you have seen in photographs, and images that can somehow surface from unconscious memories if given time.
  - baby
  - toddler (about 3–4 years old)
  - child (about 8–10 years old)
  - now.
- Select a sandplay symbol or two that goes with each age.
- Arrange the symbols in the circle you have drawn in the way they relate to each other.
- Choose a partner or form a trio.
- Talk about these stages of your life.
- Draw the symbols on to the circle.

- Write a word under each that sums up the main feeling about each stage.

5 Tuning in with touch

- Work in pairs. One person will be the receiver, one the giver.
- The leader gives an overview of what will happen.
- Discuss your response to the idea of touch.
- Play some gentle, flowing music in the background.
- The receiver lies face up on a mattress or cushions. The body position is open and relaxed, breath is slow and relaxed. Eyes closed.
- The giver sits at the receiver's head and relaxes. (Make sure your hands are warm.)
- Giver brings his/her hands slowly and consciously on to the sides of the receiver's face. Leave your hands there for a while.
- Move your hand slowly and consciously when you apply or remove your touch.
- Touch the receiver all the way down his/her body, slowly and carefully, in silence.
- The receiver does nothing but receive and watch or listen inside.

To complete this exercise (when the giver has touched the receiver's feet) the receiver can share verbally and/or on a body outline drawing what he/she felt inside and any changes noted.

Exercises for support groups

Throughout this book there are many exercises that prompt and promote personal healing. Many are ideal for exploring in a group setting. Integration of the insights and experiences engendered by working with the exercises can often take place more effectively within a group.

To choose the exercises that could form the focus of support group exploration turn to the Index of Journal Questions and Exercises on page 192.

These exercises should be woven into a programme that is agreed on by the group and should follow these basic stages:

- Developing trust — with each other and with the exercises
- Self-exploration
- Dealing with feelings — emotional release if needed
- Integration through discussion, drawing, dance and/or writing
- Support for new creativity and any follow up work.

Cycles in the journey

In reviewing your work with a support group you may perceive that your journey is cyclical. There will be times when you seem to return to a familiar place. These are transition periods. Cycles are moving, alive, and spiralling!

When your inner healing journey is truly supported you will go through periods of clearsightedness. These periods may well be followed by a strong ego reaction because you are moving from living in illusion to facing reality. There is a cycle of breaking down of ego-strength leading to surrender to inner life and inner direction. We sometimes go over familiar ground in our inner work, but see it from a more mature perspective.

As you grow up you can begin to feel yourself moving from blaming others to owning your part in creating your life. There is the cycle of moving from victim beliefs to hero(ine) actions; moving from searching for support and safety to finding inner resources; from seeking love to loving. And of course we sometimes feel like the cycle is going the other way!

There is always an ongoing cycle of uncovering previously repressed emotional pain, or memories, to feeling the pain and expressing it, and being clear again. This spiral of cycles brings hope and proof that deep change is possible.

The horizon of what is possible for us always widens. Our expectations grow and seek new distant horizons. The inner child can latch on to this natural aspect of your inner quest and use it as proof that there is no progress, and that old negative beliefs are true.

The questions for the serious journeyer will often be:

- How can I consciously make these transitions, cycle after cycle, over and over, until they are deeply known to my organism?
- How can I make these transitions consciously until they really are transformations?

For example, how often will we remember to move from anxiety to excitement; from depression to discovering and releasing what is depressed; from confusion to recognising the difficult choice between two possibilities? How often will we recognise that we have regressed to a childish state and then see and take the missed adult steps? It is important to recognise these four basic cycles. They will probably constitute your inner work for a long time.

Gradually, your inner healer will help you select aspects of your inner world that you are ready to heal at a deeper level or in more detail. Working on, or with, the transitions that appear through these cycles, results in transformation and permanent changes.

A group, or at least a co-journeyer, is extremely helpful, if not essential in enabling you to recognise these cycles and break free to move on.

Ending work with a support group

This journey is about reclaiming yourself, becoming yourself more fully and more truly. This is a state without projections, without the inner child running the show, without contraction in the body, without deadness of feelings, without unfounded and limiting beliefs in the mind.

In the journey of life each of us has to leave the parental home at some stage. This is our original centre, we are part of the parents' centre of gravity. We have to leave and create our own centre, our own energy field. Frequently we resist this. Leaving a support group or a long association with a counsellor is similar. You may need the connection long enough to establish your own inner centre, your own inner support, but then this is taken out into the world.

Jung says that if we fail to cut the child/parent ties and any later re-creations of this, and if we don't create our own authentic lives, we will regress in our development. Not leaving, not moving on, will hold up your progress towards individuation.

Do we want this responsibility? It is easier to say 'I need to belong' and act this out throughout life. Don't be afraid of feeling the end of something good. Although you will miss the energy that linked the group, you have created your own strength through deep and honest sharing, openness, freedom to be vulnerable.

There are several ways of coping with endings. Psychological and emotional withdrawal is a common way of actually leaving before facing the external separation. Some people begin to criticise the group or counsellor like teenagers ready to leave home, finding faults with parents. Other people make new plans so that technically there is no ending. The healthy way involves a clear and straightforward feeling of the ending.

Support groups will benefit from a definite lifespan and regular review of purpose and direction. Make the ending conscious by ritualising and celebrating the gains from working with the group.

5

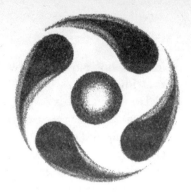

Maps, Methods and Mentors
GROUP HEALING WORK

An expert facilitator prepares participants properly with
thorough information. She creates and maintains an
environment conducive to deep surrender and exploration.
An able facilitator allows and moves with the participants'
experience without superimposing her own assumptions or
interpretations.

Kylea Taylor from *The Breathwork Experience* (1994)

Reclaiming your unconscious

Recognising your shadow and reclaiming its treasure

Self-discovery and healing work will eventually open you to
seeing your shadow. This entails recognising previously
unconscious aspects of yourself that are not usually liked or
approved of. Working with a support group is one of the best
ways to promote this work of eliminating the shadow and
reclaiming its treasure. 'Shadow' is Jung's word for the hidden
aspects of personality that have probably brought you trouble
and separation rather than love and approval. Facing your
shadow can be quite shocking but your reaction begins new
work of acknowledging all that the persona, the developing

ego, has pushed away or placed in the garbage bin — with the lid firmly on!

All that is pushed away, hidden, not lived, not expressed — yet is truly there — forms your shadow. This includes hate, rage and malice, and possibly the full passion of your love and sexuality. For many people the highest levels of their positive potential and spirituality have also been relegated to the shadow.

Remember that the unconscious elements of your psyche have a great deal of power to direct and often sabotage your life. Also, holding the contents of your shadow in the unconscious takes a lot of energy. So the aim in exploring the shadow is to release and integrate its contents and reclaim its energy for your daily living.

Becoming familiar with your ego mechanisms allows you to access and acknowledge some of your shadow aspects, clearing the way for you to hear a more subtle voice inside. Perhaps this inner guide is the voice of your soul. In any case it really knows more about living in a way that is replenishing, and can act as a link between your personal self and the highest, spiritual Self. But before this subtle stage, comes the reclaiming of the lifeforce, the fuel for growth, that has been locked away with all that is unacceptable. It is this stage that calls for even more willingness to face your truth and accept that you may not be the person you have been telling yourself — and everyone else — that you are.

If you open to the shadow in your unconscious you usually find yourself opening to fear as well. It is very disturbing to discover unseen facets of your personality but it is better to know where your 'danger' lies and where so much of your energy is held, rather than being hostage to the unpredictable breaking out of your unconscious shadow.

Realising that much of your treasure also lies in the depth of the unconscious is an incentive to explore more and more. Gradually nothing much else really matters! Your task becomes the challenge to make the shadow conscious and then to let it integrate with your day-to-day consciousness.

Living in 'search mode' causes an internal friction. Knowing the inner truth chafes at the image we see ourselves constantly presenting. This friction, if you don't resist, awakens your conscience to be true to yourself. An inner sense grows, 'I must be true, no matter what!' But at this point you may begin to fear that in recognising the shadow you will become its victim!

It is certainly true that in giving yourself permission to be real, to own more of the shadow, you will find that what had been locked away can burst forth like a wild animal caged too long. But after this transition time the energy of the 'darkness' blends with the light, the shadow becomes integrated, you feel more real, more whole. Those close to us, of course, may have to adjust as well!

No one can become conscious of the shadow without a conscious effort which challenges the whole ego, the personality. It takes courage to acknowledge the dark aspects of the ego as existing active forces.

Luckily the shadow is not the whole of the unconscious personality. It is made up of our unknown or little known attributes and qualities. Whether the shadow becomes your friend or enemy depends largely upon yourself. These hidden parts seem hostile only when ignored, forbidden or misunderstood.

Sometimes, though not often, an individual lives out the worst side of his or her nature, and represses the better side. In such cases, the shadow appears as a positive figure. But to people who live out their natural positive emotions and qualities, the shadow may appear as cold and negative.

The shadow will usually be filled with the qualities that we find we most dislike in others. Your unconscious effort to hold at bay certain qualities (e.g. meanness, jealousy, selfishness etc.) will make you project them on to others. These 'others' may in fact have some of these qualities, but we usually load them with ours as well! After we load others with what is really inside us, we find ourselves reacting strongly to them.

Since for most of us the shadow contains valuable and vital forces, it needs to be exposed and integrated, not battled against. Also, if anything is held down in us, to some degree, everything is held down.

Joseph Campbell, the great twentieth-century mythologist, says: 'Our interpretation of the word demon as meaning the demonic is very interesting. The demonic comes from the Greek, and it refers to the dynamic of life — your demon is the dynamic of life.'

In self-discovery exercises and in dreams your unconscious may sometimes present you with symbols of your shadow. These may be devils, devouring animals, dark eyes, or scenes of destruction. Very occasionally, in someone deeply split from the shadow, the shadow energy seems to manifest as a separate entity. The notion of possession by evil spirits arises from an unacceptable yet powerfully emerging shadow. For people new to self-discovery work this idea may be frightening, but with experience we realise these symbols, or so-called 'entities' are heralding new life, integration and wholeness. Then any anxiety about exploring your inner world really becomes excitement.

It can be helpful to give your shadow images a context. For example, a study of comparative mythology, folklore, religion and alchemy can help you link up with similar patterns in others through the ages. Mythology and folklore have provided warnings about the shadow and graphically shown what happens when it takes over. This is similar to the contemporary fascination with the shadow in popular cinema and literature.

The fact that recognition of your unconscious reality involves honest self-examination, and inevitably some re-organisation of life, will cause many people to drop their healing journey. It takes 'guts and determination' to pursue life by confronting the unconscious seriously. To be whole means to be aware of your opposites, your shadow, and your projections. Note the difference between awareness and acting on it. It is said we should be aware of our shadow, or beware of it!

To integrate all the facets of your psyche requires that you show yourself the same kindness and understanding you would give your friends and family. You need to take responsibility for yourself and allow your self-image to adjust as you reclaim what has been projected out on to others, on to the world. Only complete honesty will be productive and lead to the freedom you long for.

Steps to integrating the shadow energy

These steps may be explored individually in your journal writing, but they will be more effective in the context of a trusted support group. The exercise may be directed by a leader or facilitator, with participants working in pairs, taking turns at the inner exploration. It is ideal to work with a group that is accustomed to and comfortable with emotional upset and expression.

Step 1

Get in touch with yourself.
• Lie down, take some deep breaths, relax.
• Really feel what is going on inside.

Step 2

Align yourself with your shadow for a while.
• Think about what it contains or hides. What are you asked to deny in daily life? Share this.
• Imagine playing out, or living out, the parts of the shadow that are opposite to your usual self—knowing that you would not actually have to do this—to reclaim the energy that was invested in the hiding.

Step 3

Allow your body to feel the energy that would come from not hiding anything, from reclaiming your full potential. Note any fear of this. Share what you experience.

Step 4

Reflect on who you really are with the shadow side as well as the ideal side. Establish an accurate self-image.

Step 5

Share with the group, or write down in your personal journal, what you have learned about your unconscious.

Release from the idealised self-image

Your spiritual self cannot be freed unless you learn to feel all your feelings, unless you learn to accept every part of your being no matter how destructive it may be right now. No matter how negative, mean, vain, or egotistical you may find a corner of yourself to be — contrary to other, more developed aspects of your personality — it is absolutely necessary that every aspect of your being be accepted and dealt with.

Eva Pierrakos from *The Pathwork of Self-Transformation*

It is your idealised self-image — or mask self — that often prevents you knowing the shadow and claiming your wholeness. An idealised self-image is originally created as a means of attaining life, happiness, security and self-confidence. It was what you strived for so that you would feel loved. The child quickly strove to find the right image and then live up to it. The stronger the idealised self-image, the more genuine self-confidence fades away. Since in following this image you are always being other than your true self you have no real emotional or psychological security.

A longing develops in your early years for acceptance of your true self. We all long to have our true self recognised by those around us. At the same time we have smothered this true self with our effort to be ideal. There is always some acceptance and achievement associated with the idealised self so we feel we cannot risk dropping the mask. But of course our true situation remains unfulfilling.

You can recognise the idealised self-image at work when you feel failure, frustration, compulsion, guilt, shame, humiliation, strain and tension. Holding on to an idealised self-image creates a 'climate' of control in our personality. Striving for enhancement of idealised self-image leads to increased estrangement from real self. Giving it up brings a strong sense of liberation.

SELF-DISCOVERY EXERCISE
Exploring the idealised self-image

This is a good exercise to explore in pairs as part of a group experience. It can also bring much insight as a solo journal exercise. It should only be attempted in a group where there has been some bonding and a development of trust.

1 Focus

Decide which is the most important aspect of your life. For example:

- your job/career
- life with your children
- your relationship/friendships
- community life
- your inner journey.

(At some stage all these areas could be explored.)

2 The ideal

Ponder, share, write about and explore your ideal in this area — the ideal you. Consider how your feelings, body attitudes, beliefs, actions, spiritual outlooks should be to fit this ideal.

3 The actual

Consider, share, write your assessment of the real current situation. Look for any aspects that cause you to have a sense of failure, guilt, shame or strain.

4 The shadow

What do you suspect is in the shadow? What underlying negative or destructive impulses, thoughts or feelings do you have to guard against? What impulses or urges threaten the ideal?

5 Freedom

Visualise your life free from this strain. Be open to a sense of liberation in admitting to the shadow aspects and a sense of relief in letting go of the ideal. Let your body respond in any way it would like.

Projection

Give compassion and acceptance to each other in group work — and those around you in daily life. This is a key to your growth. In fact, most sacred texts demand this of seekers, often with little guidance on achieving it. Naturally, it is an easy task when you like another person and find their personality acceptable. Inevitably though you will find many people more difficult to work with. This is often due to the characteristics you project on to them as well as the projections they place on you. These projections can be a barrier to real connection and understanding.

A projection is a trait, attitude, feeling, or a piece of behaviour which actually belongs to your own personality but is not experienced as such. Instead, it is attributed to objects or persons in the environment and then experienced as directed toward you by them. The projector, unaware for instance that he or she is rejecting others, believes that other people are rejecting him or her.

The mechanism of projection happens unconsciously. It interrupts mounting pressure or excitement that we cannot cope with. This is how it can work:

1 You have an impulse, say, aggression.
2 You unconsciously interrupt the expression of the impulse, (you don't realise that you are aggressive).
3 You exclude it from expression (you hold the aggression in).
4 You become aware that it exists, and deduce that it must come from the outside, (you think the world is full of aggressive people).
5 It seems to be out there directed towards you.

Since projection is an unconscious mechanism, don't blame yourself. You simply need to recognise that the impulse happens, and then acknowledge the projection, search for the source within you, and reclaim what is inside. You will recognise a projection by the strength of your reaction.

Prejudice is an important and dangerous class of projection. Negative traits which are attributed to groups of people really belong to the prejudiced person, but this awareness is repressed. A tendency or trait that you refuse to admit in yourself (e.g. prejudices, snobbishness, prudishness, meanness) may lead you to feel indignation at that trait (real or imagined) in another.

We project on to people who are appropriate screens, that is, who manifest enough of a particular trait or attitude to make it easy for us to justify loading them with our share of it as well. Disowned qualities and emotions are projected out, unconsciously, and then felt as coming to us, not from us. This happens with both negative and positive qualities.

Examples of disowned qualities that may be projected out:
• Unacknowledged excitement is felt as anxiety — something 'out there' seems to be making us anxious.

- Your desire and drive are felt as pressure.
- Your aggression is felt as fear.
- Your anger is felt as depression.
- Your own unrecognised potential is projected out and comes back to you as a sense of over-blown awe at other people's achievements.

In other words you are responsible for the anxiety, the pressure, the fear, the awe, you experience.

How can we tell if what we sense in another is really them or our projection? Ken Wilbur, in *No Boundary*, sums it up like this: 'If it is purely something about them we feel informed. If it is a projection we feel affected.'

SELF-DISCOVERY EXERCISE
Using projections to know yourself

Again this exercise can be an individual or group experience. In group work, participants can work in pairs, one listening and encouraging the exploration, the other doing the exercise and sharing what is found.

1 Think of someone you fear. Tell your partner or write:
   'What I fear in you (this person you are thinking of) is ...'
   'What I fear in myself is ... (repeat same thing)'
   Give yourself time to feel it inside, then see if there is any truth in the similarity.
2 Think of someone you really disapprove of. Tell your partner, or write:
   'What I disapprove of in you is ...'
   'What I disapprove of in myself is ... (same thing)'
   Give yourself time to feel it inside, then see if there is any truth in the similarity.
3 Think of the person you most admire. Tell your partner, or write:
   'What I admire in you is ...'
   'What I admire in myself is ... (same thing).'
   Give yourself time to feel it inside, then see if there is any truth in the similarity.
4 Think of someone who is strong in a way that you admire. Tell your partner, or write:

'The strength I see in you is ...'

'The strength I await in myself is ... (same thing).'

Give yourself time to feel it inside, then see if there is any truth in the similarity.

Review what you have thought about and written. Now share it with a support person or write down:

- your main insights
- how the exercise has left you feeling
- a sense of areas in yourself you need to explore further
- some steps that will help you explore further.

Transference

The dictionary definition of transference is: 'A psycho-analytical term. The patient transfers his own emotions on to the analyst, for example, he may develop an intense love or hatred of him. Also used if the patient transfers his own emotions on to someone else as when he blames someone else for what he has done himself.' *Faber Medical Dictionary*.

This mechanism not only operates regularly in daily life but also in group interaction when we focus on inner healing. Transference was discovered and described by the early psychoanalysts. It is most important to recognise and reclaim projections and transferences because they rob us of clarity and intensity of experience.

Transference is a specific form of projection. It is the unconscious assignment of feelings and attitudes to other people in the present that were originally associated with important figures (parents, siblings, etc.) in one's early life.

When working in or with a group, some of the participants' feelings for their parents may be transferred to you, especially if you are a group leader. This transference may be negative or positive. Neither positive nor negative transference is desirable but certainly negative transference feels less comfortable than positive. It is necessary to work with these feelings and expose the transference so that group relationship can begin to deepen.

Freud spoke of the inevitable transference of the childhood fixation to the analyst in order to work through it to the actual situation. In group work it can also be therapeutic when transference is discovered, discussed and taken back.

Transference was a major tool in the early analytical schools, since childhood experiences were not available directly, but could be deduced by watching the transference in the relationship to the therapist. Emotional Release Counselling activates and directly contacts childhood material and releases it in safe, constructive ways.

Transference should not be criticised. It happens unconsciously and needs to be recognised and used productively, that is, processed in relation to people from the past.

People transfer on to group leaders, therapists, gurus, spouses, children, friends, groups, governments, God, material objects — anything and anybody at all. There is no blame attached to either transferee or transferor for this phenomenon. It is natural for the psyche to try to complete unfinished business from the past.

Transference largely comes from the hurt inner child, so we need to support each other in group work in being alert to the inner child and its reactions. In a supported situation, it is possible for the adult you to allow the hurt inner child to feel deeply the painful childhood experiences and thus let them heal. The child is allowed and encouraged to take centre stage in this process time, and re-live, re-feel its needs, its aloneness, its despair, its rage and hatred, its love and vulnerability.

The activation of projection and transference is the main reason why some healing groups may break up or stagnate, or even degenerate and actually become destructive. Having some expertise on hand to deal with these two psychic processes in group work is ideal, and the input of a trained facilitator is extremely valuable.

Body focus

The body, energy and emotional release

In a healthy person, energy and emotions are meant to flow together through the body. When they are bottled up or blocked we feel unhealthy, or unwhole. A measure of the success of your healing journey is the free flowing of energy and feelings. This flow is your lifeforce. It is impossible to feel very alive and have dead emotions. You cannot be very alive and be holding in one particular feeling, or block off one thing from the past. So for full aliveness in your body — the home of your feelings and energy — you need to release held-in emotions and free up static lifeforce.

Emotional growth and healing requires body, feelings and mind to come together, to reconnect. The disconnection has resulted from repression of hurts, disappointments, anger and traumas from the past. When these parts are reconnected your emotional pain will be released. Emotional pain is often unconscious and stored away in the body. It may become visible through physical pain which is often a signpost that emotions are buried beneath. Tension in the body is often the result of your energy being diverted or dammed up from its natural flow or expression. Underneath physical pain and tension is emotional pain and positive energy.

Much of the ERC understanding of the body/energy/ emotions connection comes from experiential exploration of the ideas and approaches of Dr Wilhelm Reich. His work spans the three levels of psychology and supports our search from personal healing to spiritual awakening.

Body armouring

The blockage of emotions and energy which you feel in tight muscles is called armouring. A chronic problem of tension may correspond with a record of past trauma. Wilhelm Reich wrote that, 'The body is frozen history'.

ERC work may begin with a focus on the body's symptoms. Try to adopt a readiness to open yourself to feeling the life of the body. Your training may be to occupy yourself with thoughts and fantasies and to alternate this with what is happening in the outer world. There are not many people who have developed a good connection with the life of the body, or an understanding of the body's language and the meaning of its symptoms.

To explore and let the body be free we use strong breath. This brings in the energy we need to make internal connections. Touch is often used to focus the body, to anchor awareness within. Then you need to practise listening to the body. Listen for any memories stored in the body, or any messages it may give through released feelings, or imagery, or impulses to move in a certain way.

The exploration of body energy is carried out with an attitude of surrender which you need to allow an ego shift and to let go of your defences. Surrendering means you consciously agree to feel any old or difficult feelings that may be stored within. Your new willingness to feel and express yourself opposes the hurt inner child's learned way of repression. Then with your feelings and body energy alive you are supported to move or release or become still, to follow exactly what the body knows — in its wisdom — needs to happen for your healing.

Many people fear being too alive. This fear can be conscious or unconscious and may be reflected in mistrust of the body, its urges, its excitement. It is a problem that can begin at birth (fear of hurting mother), be reinforced in childhood (we are told to be quiet and still, and to hide our truth), and often becomes chronic in adulthood (our effort to fit in and be good becomes a habit).

There are seven main segments of armouring in the body. In these segments the organs and tissue work together to hold or protect us against difficult feelings and energies, or to release and allow energy flow. These areas of the body respond with a basic 'yes' or 'no'. When an energy current cannot run up and down the body as it should because it is obstructed by armour blocks, a sideways movement results which, means 'no'.

In *The Function of the Orgasm* (1973) Wilhelm Reich describes the segments of armouring as the organs and muscle groups which have functional contact with one another and which are capable of accompanying each other in what he called 'the emotional expressive movement'. From his research he describes the armour segments as having a horizontal structure, never vertical (except the arms and legs). Segments are arranged at right angles to the spine. He describes energy currents and emotions flowing parallel to the body axis.

The seven segments identified by Wilhelm Reich are:
1 Ocular — Eyes, forehead, ears, nose, back of skull

2 Oral — lips, chin, jaws, throat, occipital muscles (back of head)
3 Cervical — neck, throat, tongue
4 Thoracic — chest, intercostals, shoulders, arms, hands
5 Diaphragmatic — diaphragm, stomach, solar plexus
6 Abdominal — abdominal muscle, ribs to pelvis
7 Pelvic — muscles of pelvis, thigh, buttocks, genitals, legs, feet.

The seven segments relate to the positions of the seven chakras and associated nerve plexuses. Releasing blocks in segments increases flow of lifeforce through the body and allows chakras to come into action. Chakras are potential focuses of strong energy. Their function is the reception and distribution of energy through the body and beyond. De-armouring is the first essential step in the work that can eventually open us to spiritual energy.

ERC body focus work is designed to help people become more aware and connected to their body. All group work should include exercises to enhance this awareness. It is your inner connection, along with the physical and emotional release of armouring, that brings real health to the energy flow. A healthy energy flow creates a more balanced and positive emotional state, and is a preparation for spiritual — or spirited — energy.

There are three layers of the personality that relate to body energy:

1 Mask self — facade or social veneer, supported by our idealised self-image;
2 Secondary layer — underlying negativity — rage, hate, malice, contempt (shadow qualities). This layer relates to the armouring;
3 The core — always healthy and flowing, wanting to expand. Reich describes it as running through the centre of the body.

Reich says: 'Inhibited pleasure is transformed into rage, and inhibited rage is transformed into muscular spasm'. Rage is a forceful push of energy occurring when the natural soft flow is blocked. It is most important for us to mobilise and allow safe expression of hate. We need to convert hate and rage into love and caring. Most of us need deep healing work on this secondary layer to find how to let our bodies and feelings go from hard to soft, cold to warm. It is work which most of us secretly wish we could avoid!

There are four basic stages in opening up the personality and the body. Group work can help:

1 Penetrate the mask self. In a group everyone can practise being their real self.
2 Release the secondary layer or lower self. Underlying emotional negativity and physical armouring is most effectively neutralised through emotional release processing work (see page 158).
3 Connect with the core, or Higher Self. Letting your core energy flow outwards may involve stillness, relaxation, meditation or sometimes strong dance. To help the core energy flow out, to express itself, may mean that you really throw yourself into your outer life for a while.
4 Find new direction for your outer life from this contact. Allow your outer life to follow the inner life. This involves gradually recognising your purpose and the contribution to the world that your life can make.

The pulse of the universe is expansion and contraction. The same pulsing is in you. Your lifetime aim should be to avoid becoming fixed in a contracted state. Often deep release methods and powerful free dance will reveal how contracted your body, energy and feelings are. Group gatherings provide good times for strong dance. Once you taste expansion, and also see the possibilities in the work of your co-journeyers, your motivation for the healing journey is strengthened.

There is a relationship between your personal expansion and your reception of lifeforce, the cosmic energy. Another parallel exists between your psychic and muscular contraction and the continuation of your negative emotions. Ongoing group work can inspire you and give you the determination to overturn old limiting habits of contraction.

Some of the aims and stages of ERC work, with and through the body, include:

• Allowing the mask self to drop away.
• Clearing fear of aliveness.
• Releasing personal reasons (from the past) for blocking feelings and energy.

- Allowing armouring to soften.
- Converting negative energy into flowing positivity.
- Re-establishing the 'yes' flow through the body segments.
- Allowing core energy to flow outwards and be expressed.
- Living your life wholeheartedly; using your core energy in daily life.
- Allowing lifeforce to awaken chakras and subtle spiritual energies.
- Finding out who you really are and what you have to offer.

Emotional anatomy

Different parts of the body tend to hold on to particular feelings. Each seeker needs to explore their own body symptoms and learn what is held in each area of armouring. The following list is simply a guide to what many find. Hopefully, having a few clues to commonly held feelings will support your insights and understanding. Remember body pains, tensions or blocks can be the doorways to release and healing, so we work to achieve a deeper and more friendly relationship with the sensations of the body.

Forehead:	Denial. Not wanting to know something or see the truth.
Eyes:	Sadness, incomplete grieving, tears.
Jaw:	Anger, words held in or bitten back.
Neck:	Control, not wanting to surrender.
Shoulders:	The weight of being and feeling controlled or nagged.
Back:	Upper: Locked up grief, the will to achieve. Lower: The need for, or lack of, support.
Chest:	Grief, longing, loss.
Arms, hands:	Expression, creativity. Holding back from hitting out. Wanting to reach out.
Diaphragm:	Deep sobbing.
Belly:	Fear and/or excitement.
Buttocks:	Anger, rage, hate.
Thighs:	Outside: Unexpressed power, latent strength. Inside: Unfulfilled sexuality, sensuality.
Knees:	Flexibility, resistance to growing up.

Release of armouring

Some approaches to dissolving armouring should only be attempted with a professional emotional release counsellor or Reichian-trained therapist. The very best way for many people is through transpersonal breathwork.

Often in breathwork sessions it is as if the inner healer finds the body's tense areas, the blockages, and momentarily increases them and at the same time increases your awareness and sensitivity to them, until understanding and release follow. Breathwork will promote long-term freedom from armouring.

Once your deep tension is released the bands of armouring relax. While new ways of being and behaving may take time, exploration and practice to develop, the old restrictions will not be able to take over again.

Bioenergetics is a set of physical movements devised by Dr Alexander Lowen and Dr John Pierrakos, colleagues and students of Wilhelm Reich. The exercises are designed to activate held-in emotions and stir up the energy flow of the body. Some exercises are quite emotionally expressive and can trigger strong feelings. An ERC facilitator is trained to use these exercises to support your healing. Combining prescribed movements with rhythm and dance work is an enjoyable way to work free of armouring.

De-armouring and bioenergetics begins with the eyes and face and works down the body. The exercises start lightly at the skin and then work gradually, more deeply, in towards the core.

Armouring will really only give way fully when the emotions underneath are fully felt and released, so that there are no longer any held-in emotions to armour against. This takes professional support because most of what is underneath is buried in the unconscious.

However, you have begun the search for more aliveness already and you have taken responsibility for your own journey. Here are some ways that you can support your own de-armouring. Do these exercises with a deep self-awareness. Listen to your body; don't force it. Surrender to whatever happens.

- Relax with slow deep breathing for short periods.
- Massage yourself.
- Explore strong facial expressions. Practise making faces that go with strong emotions, and add sounds (e.g. move from a fearful face to an angry face; from sad face to happy face).
- Make strong sounds (e.g. shouting, animal noises, humming, singing).
- Tense yourself and hold the tension for a short time. Intentionally use muscular stress to help de-armouring and allow vibration to develop in the muscles.

Vibration is nature's way of releasing stress. Some bioenergetics exercises are the most helpful here. Refer to Alexander and Leslie Lowen *The Vibrant Way to Health*. This excellent book, which is a manual of bioenergetics, is out of print but can be found in libraries.

BODY AWARENESS EXERCISE
Body focus

This simple Gestalt and massage approach is ideal for group work. The aim is to listen more deeply to the unconscious in your body and to connect with physical pain or holding. You may hear an emotional message that has been locked in the body. The exercise needs to be treated as a very precious time to 'listen' to the wisdom of your body in whatever way it may speak.

- Work in pairs.
- One person (the seeker) lies down on their back in a relaxed, open position (not curled up), on thick carpet, cushions or mattress.
- The other person sits at the seeker's head and listens.
- Gentle music in the background gives privacy and promotes surrender.

Seeker's instructions
- Become aware of your breath, allow it to expand.
- Check through inside from head to toes.
- Let some part call your attention — some part that is 'troublesome', in pain, stressed or is filled with a very strong energy.

- Tell your partner, the listener, about it.
- Put your hand or the listener's hand on the part. (Turn on your side if the part is at your back.) The touch is an anchor for your awareness.
- Listen to the questions that are about to be asked of that part.
- Let your ego surrender. Let the part hear and respond.
- Let that part use your voice to answer, so that your listener can hear.
- Take a full breath after each question.

Guided questions for the listener to slowly ask

1 Are you something new, or old; something ancient or recent?
2 Are you deep or on the surface?
3 Are you in the bones or tissues? Maybe in the muscles or skin?
4 Are you a tight, holding energy or diffuse?
5 Have you got a shape? Describe your shape and size. (Go right inside that part. Become the part totally and take time to listen deeply.)
6 What colour are you? Be specific and describe the subtleties.
7 Is the energy still or vibrating?
8 Did somebody else cause you? Or the person whose body you are in?
9 Do you have a name?
10 Do you have a sound?
11 Is there anything you stop the person doing?
12 What do you want of the person whose body you are in? What do you want them to do for you?
13 Is there somewhere you'd like to move to?
14 Is there anything you would like to say to the rest of the body?
15 Would this part like some massage?
16 Breathe and open to any image or memory. Be with that for a while; allow any movement or change in body position.
17 Is there anything else the part would like to make known?
18 Come into the whole of yourself now, as well as the part.

- Listener removes touch gently.
- Share insights. Discuss these questions:
    - Has the sensation changed? In what way?
    - How easy or difficult did you find the exercise?
    - Were you aware of any resistance or distractions?
    - How do you feel now?
- The seeker draws a mandala or expresses the experience on a body outline.

SELF-AWARENESS QUESTIONS
What am I holding under the armouring?

Gaining insight into the inner meanings of particular areas of armouring can be a great help in self-understanding. But remember that your psyche works in a unique way so this exercise is a guide only for your own questioning, research and discovery. Always take the time to reach your own self-awareness; don't just believe in the list!

Instructions:

- Lie down and relax. Take some full breaths. Let go of the outside world.
- Tune in to any pains, aches or parts of the body that are calling out in any way.
- Stay focussed on them for a few minutes.
- In your mind, ask the part to reveal the emotional expression held there, then write it down.
- Read what is on the list below and compare it to what you found.
- Give yourself time with your journal for further insights and new directions to emerge.
- Ponder:
    - 'How does my inner experience and the phrases below relate to my life now? My life in the past?'
    - 'What do I need to come to further wholeness?'

Head: I don't want to know about what is happening in my life.
I'm confused. It's too much!
I don't want to know the source of my pain.

Eyes:	I won't let you see me cry.
	Can't you see me? See me! You never, never saw me!
	I won't look at it. I couldn't bear to see what was happening.
Jaw:	I can't say what I mean. I won't!
	I have to hold it back. If I said what I mean you would never love me again (or) you'll hit me.
	I don't know what to say.
Neck:	You're a pain in the neck!
	I have to swallow my feelings/reactions/tears/ anger.
	Yes/no (confusion)
	I can't let this energy come right up because it gets me into trouble.
Chest:	If I hold my breath I won't feel the pain.
	My heart is breaking. I'll never give in.
	I'll never let you in. You broke my heart.
Shoulders and arms:	I have to hold back from smashing you in the face.
	I have to hold back from reaching out to you.
	Don't hold me down.
Chest and arms:	Please hold me. I want you. I need you.
	Where are you (mummy/daddy)? I'm only little.
	Touch me/don't touch me. Don't let me go.
	Keep them (the bad people) away from me.
Shoulders and back:	Get off my back! You load me down.
	You're always holding me down and now I do it to myself!
	It's all too much — the load is too big.
Diaphragm:	I'll never fully feel. The gate is locked!
	I'll never let you in. I'll never let my feelings up.
	I'm really scared to feel/to let anyone in.
Belly:	You make me feel sick. You are sick!
	I get knotted up when I think of you!
	I'm afraid!
Pelvis and buttocks:	I hate you so much!
	I'll never let you see how much I hate.
	I'm hurting, don't hurt me.

Legs: You took my stand from me. I can't keep up.
            I could kick you in the face. I hate your power over me.
            There's nothing I can depend on.

SELF-AWARENESS QUESTIONS
What lies under the surface of body pains?

This exercise is a follow-up to 'What am I holding under the armouring?' on page 155. The questions below will help you probe any further possible emotional components that may be just under the surface of your consciousness. It is through questioning, listening and connecting to what is really there inside you that emotional release and de-armouring occurs.

Forehead: Is there something I don't want to know?
            What have I stopped myself thinking about?
            Am I controlling my temper with my thoughts?
            Am I 'thinking' a hurt away (rationalising)?

Eyes: Did I try to stop myself crying?
            Was I afraid to see something?
            Am I too embarrassed to show how I feel?

Neck: Is it very hard always holding myself up?
            Has someone been nagging me?
            Am I controlling my energy all the time?
            Do I stop my 'no' or my 'yes'?

Jaw: What do I really need to say?
            Do I always want to win?
            When did I bite back those angry words?

Shoulders   Who has been 'on my back'?
and upper   Whose load am I really carrying?
back: Am I afraid to be 'up front' about something?

Chest: What am I really longing for?
            Who doesn't want me?
            Who am I closed off from?

Elbows   Who do I want to hug?
and wrists: Who do I want to push away?
            What creative thing do I want to do but am not doing?

Belly:	Who am I afraid of?
	Who makes me sick?
	What excitement did I try to hide?
Buttocks	What anger am I hiding?
and lower	Is it dangerous to really hate someone?
back:	Have I ignored my sexual feelings?
	What is the risk in being strong and powerful?
Ankles	Who left me suddenly?
and calves:	Is it hard to keep up?
	What do I have to hold on to with great strength?
	Would I like to run away?
Knees:	Do I resist changes?
	Am I afraid of growing?

Emotional release processes

Some of us are so defended against unpleasant memories and feelings in the unconscious that we need to focus more directly on releasing these defences before the work with symbols and body focus can be helpful. An array of triggering mechanisms is used by trained ERC facilitators to bring up the repressed material — this is called processing. It is usually done with an experienced or trained group or counsellor. The methods can also be applied to individual release work with professional support.

By connecting with and totally accepting your feelings, you may work back through the past to basic emotional and behavioural imprints. These patterns from the past may be contributing to dysfunctional or destructive behaviour in the present. Once you have identified old imprints you can then work with them, fully feel them, express and release them from your psyche.

The energy, focus and inspiration of a group is ideal for processing and emotional release. Since many inner stories are similar and because hurts have a similar source, watching others confront their feelings may be a catalyst for you. Observing other people will greatly accelerate your own healing work by touching memories and feelings that have been well hidden. In a group there is much more energy and emotional support for venturing inside ourselves. There is also the gift of observing another in their vulnerability. We see our fellow journeyers break through their usual reserve, drop through the layers of anger, rage, hate, grief and arrive in a tender new space of love and self-acceptance.

Processing deals very much with both current reactions and the hurt inner child. It can lead to clear insights about the non-productive patterns in your life. The various processing methods form an important step in your journey toward emotional maturity. The more confronting approaches should only be used by trained practitioners. The effectiveness of processing methods always depends on the facilitator's skills and experience in creating trust and being able to mirror what is happening so that it can be more deeply felt. The facilitator also sets a tone, an energy field, and much depends on the depth of their experience.

An important requirement of healing work is being able to distinguish clearly between acting out feelings (being run by them) and processing them. To process is to acknowledge any current reactive feelings and in a safe place to allow them to emerge fully, feel the connection to the past, to have full expression and move on. A safe setting has a facilitator and cushions or mattresses for any strong physical release. Words and sounds must not be audible to outsiders and no one inside the group should become upset by strong emotional release. It is vital that those processing also are supported to take their reactions back to the real source within their own psyche.

Processing also implies that after the emotional release has occurred, a new positive state emerges from which new purpose and creativity flow. Through this work we all can become more feeling people: feel ourselves, feel others, feel the joy of life and feel deeply the beauty around us. Successful emotional processing means being able to follow a reaction back to its source and then feeling an energy flow direct from a source within.

Each processing exercise may have a specific aim, for example, you may wish to deal with relationship problems or release frustration with your boss. Generally though you aim to feel fully what seems to be too painful to feel now and is similar to what was too painful to feel in the past. The more directly confronting methods of emotional release can take you deep into current issues and expose and heal the links from your childhood and birth.

Your aim is to mobilise all that has been held in. Frequently you will progress from more difficult, negative emotions to the positive. For example, I could begin with frustration about a particular situation in my life. Exploring the feeling more deeply I may find layers of anger inside. In acknowledging the anger I may find some rage or hate. After the release of these strong feelings grief or sadness may follow. As this sadness is felt I may finally be able to contact some love and tenderness. The love and tenderness was always there but was covered over by the negative emotions. Processing often leads to a connection with new energy currents and perhaps to the Higher Self or essence.

The group must allow members time and space to integrate the old child's view with the new adult understanding. This support should also deal with the need to internalise the insights. Obviously you should not race out immediately and act upon the insights before integrating.

The newly emerging adult in you is free to relate, or not to relate, to everyone that you have had issues with. I encourage journeyers to bring their newly found love and freedom directly into all present relationships rather than harking back to old events. Making great efforts to forgive old hurts is not essential. Real forgiveness cannot take place until the unconscious resentments and hurts have been released.

Integration of the new energy and insights from emotional processing is supported by drawing, writing and sharing your experience. Often you will find that you wish to rest after dealing with anger or grief. Rest and sleep may form an important step in your integration after confronting emotional release processing.

EMOTIONAL RELEASE PREPARATION EXERCISE
The 'gateway' questions

This exercise is based on some beautiful words from *The Pathwork of Self-Transformation* by Eva Pierrakos. It is useful in widening your view of personal and emotional problems and beginning the practice of sharing openly. It can help determine where you should focus for future healing work. Do the exercise, as a writing exercise, with a leader reading through the text and asking the questions below.

- Gather crayons, drawing book and your journal.
- Play some gentle, quiet music in the background to support relaxation.
- Move to a comfortable position, maybe leaning against a wall with a pillow, or in a comfortable chair. Take time to let each aspect or each question reverberate inside. Hopefully, allow your writing to come from more than just the mind.
- Between each question take some full breaths and connect with your body awareness again.
- The leader of the group or the chairperson for the group time, begins by reading:
  Through the gateway of feeling your weakness lies your strength.
  Through the gateway of feeling your pain lies your pleasure and joy.
  Through the gateway of feeling your fear lies your security and safety.
  Through the gateway of feeling your loneliness lies your capacity to have fulfilment, love and companionship.
  Through the gateway of feeling your hopelessness lies true and justified hope.
  Through the gateway of accepting the lacks in your childhood lies your fulfilment now.
- The leader repeats a line of the text and asks a question (see below). Allow about four or five minutes for each question.

*Through the gateway of feeling your weakness lies your
strength.*

Open to feeling, to images that come into your mind, any
memories from the past. Feel what 'weakness' means to you.
What are, or were, your weaknesses? As you are ready begin
to write about this.

*Through the gateway of feeling your pain lies your pleasure
and joy.*

Can you sense that in your body? Can you allow yourself to
feel the main pain in the past and the main pain in your life
now? Give yourself time to remember and feel deeply. What is
your pain? Take some full breaths. Can you write from your
heart?

*Through the gateway of feeling your fear lies your security
and safety.*

Close your eyes for a moment. What are, and have been, the
main fears in your life? Write about these when you are ready.

*Through the gateway of feeling your loneliness lies your
capacity to have fulfilment, love and companionship.*

When are you in touch with your loneliness — now and in the
past? Write about this.

*Through the gateway of feeling your hopelessness lies true
and justified hope.*

Is there anything you feel hopeless about? An incident, a situation in your life now or in the past? Write whatever comes to
your mind.

*Through the gateway of accepting the lacks in your
childhood lies your fulfilment now.*

Take another deep breath. Think about the main lack in your
childhood? Are there things that happened that were not
acceptable? Write things as they come back to you.

- Allow yourself to open to a feeling or impression of what is
  waiting for you when you have released and healed all that
  you have been writing about.

- Now draw, expressing this in lines and colours. Don't think about the drawing, just let it flow out from within.
- Form into pairs or trios to share what stood out for you as the most important aspect of this exercise.

Exploring resistance

If you feel stuck with a particular issue or with your ongoing healing work the first step is to increase your awareness of any resistance. Jung tells us that the ego will always resist material coming from the unconscious, and many of us have seen that we resist any insights or steps that may point the way to large changes in our lives.

Resistance has a purpose. Although your rational minds may not pick it up, there is logic in the unconscious. Resistance is usually there to protect against some hurts in the recent or distant past. You may have to recognise that your resistance has been doing its job of protecting for a long time. It may have become a habit.

In exploring your resistance it is good to begin with the simplest, most obvious, possible reasons for resisting. For example, do you actually want to do healing work right now? Do you trust the environment, the group, the supporter? At this moment do you trust the process of your healing, or the particular modality? Are there any religious or philosophical reasons in the back of your mind for fearing the healing work?

There are many questions that may be standing in the way of going more deeply into your inner world. Although your conscious mind might be agreeing to explore, we know that the unconscious has more power. Pondering on these questions will help to disempower your resistance.

Questions to help understand resistance

- Do you have a fear of behaving in the same destructive way as someone in your past if the process work brings out your anger?
- Are you projecting your own self-criticism and judgments on to the group or the supporter?

- Do you have a very practical reason for wanting to stay 'together' right now, and not opening to feelings and memories?
- Do you have a fear that deep inner reflection might challenge your relationships?
- Do you feel resentment at having to do healing work? (Many of us carry a huge resentment that our past was not perfect, and that we have to be responsible for our own healing.)
- Are you still hoping that someone else could do your healing for you, or rescue you with some magic to take the pain away?
- Are you afraid of seeing the truth? Are you afraid of becoming responsible for yourself?
- Have you had a past experience of opening to inner life that:
  - led to a difficult outcome?
  - caused upset to those around you?
  - was not supported afterwards?
  - resulted in you feeling dysfunctional for some time?
  - attracted criticism?
  - left you feeling nauseous?

It is important to realise that resistance has more power when it is fully or partly hidden. Your aim is to decrease this power by making it conscious. Look at how the power is expressed. For example, how is it expressed in your thoughts? What phrases or words crop up? Do you hear things like 'I'm too tired', 'I'm confused' or 'Nothing will be different'.

How is the resistance expressed in your feelings? Are you fearful or angry? Where is it in your body? Which muscles or body parts hold it?

Resistance often appears in the choice of the processing topic. Is the topic you are trying to explore a red herring? What is the essential area to explore? For example, a client of mine recently suggested focussing on financial worries, when really the relationship with his wife was calling for urgent attention. The intimate relationship seemed to be falling apart, but he felt he had to explore what he called his 'poverty consciousness'. No doubt there would be a link between these two issues, but the money problem was more abstract, and less painful, to deal with.

Newly emerging resistance usually has a lot of power. Try not to increase the power of resistance by fighting it directly. After making it conscious, as described above, you could exaggerate it, or role-play it. Set up a dialogue with this energy. Find some imagery that describes it such as a wall, a locked door, a closed room.

Think about why the resistance needs to be there. This may lead to emerging memories of what it has been protecting you from. Try to befriend it. Allow your adult part to thank it for its past work and advise it that it is no longer needed; its usefulness has been superseded by your new intention to heal and grow.

For people completing intensive healing work

There are many ways to support the new insights and energy that emerge from a period of deep self-exploration. You may need these ideas when you get home — or back 'to the real world', as many say.

Take good care of yourself. Give yourself rest and relaxation during the next few days of integration. Give yourself time to know what you are feeling. We usually go through life ignoring our emotional life.

If you don't already have one, buy a personal journal and regularly write down what is happening in your inner life. This will help you review your healing work from time to time.

Record any vivid or troubling dreams that emerge. My experience is that people have more dreams, with more important content, after an emotional release workshop. These dreams can form an important basis for future healing work.

Begin a new habit of giving yourself systematic relaxation time purely for your inner self. It may be just a few minutes a few times a day, but become still, relax and allow the business of your day to drop away.

Also let yourself enjoy some dancing and exercising. Listen inside yourself. What is your energy wanting? Stillness? Rest? Movement? Strong release? Although it may be out of character, you may find your body really enjoys strong dance, shaking, singing, humming, even shouting. Your body is the gateway to your inner world. It is easy to neglect it, so organise a regular massage.

Drawing is a wonderful way to express newly emerging feelings. Display your mandalas and drawings. From time to time let your eye rove over them and see if any additional insights emerge. Add new drawings.

When you feel ready, arrange a time to do more healing work. Whether this is next week or in six months, it is helpful to the psyche to know that it has a special time ahead for exploration, when it will be listened to and honoured.

Reading, study and exploring the world of ideas may help you to understand and integrate the experiences you have had. Knowledge and your own experience will go together to increase your understanding. A wider knowledge of healing work will help you see the road ahead, the directions you need to follow next. There are many books that will help you further understand emotional release methods. You can refer to the list at the back of this book (see page 184).

A period of intensive healing work can disturb and unsettle you and leave you wondering why you started the journey in the first place. It is vital to have clear, experienced support if such times occur. Your inner space is no longer a place you know very well and because it is not yet fully healed it is not entirely comfortable. You will probably feel the conflict between the 'old' and the 'new' very keenly. This is a normal experience.

You may have lived for many, many years holding painful feelings at bay, and now you have agreed to feel them. That's fine in supportive group sessions. But afterwards, since the inner gates have been opened to the unconscious, the feelings may not conveniently close down again. You may need support to continue feeling, or find ways to accommodate emerging unconscious material without repressing it again.

Psychological and physical opening, resulting in new alive energy, is supported in workshop environments and when you are among fellow seekers. However, when you return to your old life, perhaps surrounded by people who do not value the new you, doubts and a desire to close down can take over. Change can be threatening to others who find it easier to relate in the old way. They may attempt to put you back in your old box. The energy that was felt as excitement, then turns to anxiety. This anxiety can even be encouraged by those around you because they are still afraid of their inner life and of strong aliveness. It is important to recognise this anxiety in its early stages and convert it to its natural form — aliveness and excitement. This can be done through taking a brisk walk, dancing, even just jumping up and down and shaking off the old, closed ways. If any anxiety seems persistent phone your supporter or facilitator and ask for advice. Don't blame yourself or try to handle things alone.

Realising that your life has been set up by a conditioned ego, or even totally run by your inner child and its fears, is a very positive step. However, healing work can leave you somewhere between your old rigid ways and the new, flowing, open ways of being that you have begun to experience. This is an uncomfortable place. The temptation is to return to the known no matter how much you may have tried to escape it in the past. During this transition time of the ego shift you often feel a bit out of synch. It is normal to find your old motivation no longer motivating. It can be tiring to constantly wonder who you really are, what you really want, what you should do. This questioning, while unsettling, forms the basis of your opportunity for growth.

Remembering and release of the inner child's pain gives you a clear insight into how you have lived out of the child's limited scripts, and how these scripts have prevented you from being fulfilled in your life.

After deep release work you may find you have plenty of freed, available energy, and your need to sleep may be diminished. This is normal. The question is what to do with this new energy? How can I express myself creatively? For other people, especially after the release of deep grief, long stretches of sleep are essential. Changes in sleeping patterns, whether short-term or long-term, can be expected.

Some healing processes bring a great deal of emotional, physical and energy release. Your body may sometimes feel tired, fragile or shaky for a few days. Although it may be uncomfortable it is normal during emotional release work. Take good care of yourself. Do not try to do heroic deeds after dealing with strong emotions. Give your body and psyche time to integrate and rest. Long hot baths, afternoon naps, reflection time with beautiful music, journalling and frequent drawing can all help the integrative process.

Remember major physical, mental and emotional changes may result from this inner work, so your total being must have time to integrate the changes.

Be cautious of advice from people who are not familiar with deep healing work. New ways of being are opening up for you. The old maps are not useful. The steps you have taken can lead to a wonderful journey into life. Wherever you are on your journey, each new step will benefit from the support of someone who has trod the path before you.

6

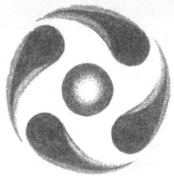

Scaling the Heights
PROFESSIONAL HEALING SUPPORT

The deep longing that exists in every human heart for a more fulfilling state of consciousness and a larger capacity to experience life must, sooner or later, impel us to look within ourselves.

Susan Thesenga from *The Undefended Self* (1994)

Choosing a counsellor

If you are in search of good professional support for your healing journey you may need to try a few counsellors or therapists before you find one you're comfortable with. In selecting a support person you should feel accepted and challenged; guided, not pushed; informed by your own insights, not instructed by the expert. Most professional counsellors have broad experience and knowledge, but counsellors that have full training in ERC will relate to you as a fellow-seeker. Professionals do not seek a superior role, and certainly they have no interest in becoming your prop, guru, or rescuer.

A good counsellor or therapist almost never interprets your experience. Gone are the days of simply handing over responsibility for your healing work to an expert. The ground-breaking work of Jung recognises that each individual psyche has its own wisdom, logic, and inbuilt way of healing and coming to individuation. An emotional release counsellor, although highly trained in experiential work in a range of modalities, is more like a fellow-seeker. Their role is to:

- help you find a starting point for your self-exploration;
- support and accompany you on your healing journey; and
- help you gain trust in your own healing process.

A counsellor who understands the ERC processes knows that prolonged intellectual analysis during healing work often turns out to be a sign of resistance and can impede your progress. They will encourage you to use your mind at the integration stage, but initially they value direct experience, listening to the body's knowledge and awareness of emotions.

An emotional release counsellor differentiates between acting out and disciplined internalisation. He or she is experienced in the psyche's avoidance, defence and resistance strategies and can guide you to feel all your emotions rather than use unconscious ploys to escape anything unpleasant.

An emotional release counsellor has participated in many hours of personal development work and they trust the way the unconscious works. They also trust your deeper wisdom, your drive towards wholeness, and can help activate that drive.

A good counsellor knows that their best strategy is to temporarily suspend all anticipation and expectations. He or she creates a neutral, accepting space and alive energy field that promotes the release of the past which is needed to heal and step forward into a positive future.

To be an effective counsellor requires a high degree of self-knowledge. Your support person must participate in the healing process without fear; and have a willingness to face new observations about themselves and their role in the process. This avoids any projection of their own fears on to you.

A counsellor should be a member of a professional association with a code of ethics and professional standards. Emotional release counsellors are required to undertake regular inservice training and supervision to promote their ongoing personal development, as well as their professional extension.

Counselling sessions

Counsellors may specialise in the methods that have given them the most help in their own journey but of course they are equipped to move through a range of methods finding how to best meet the client where they are. Whatever the main process used there are six broad stages that may be drawn from during individual sessions.

First, you and the counsellor together will look for something positive within, such as hope, inner strength or treasure. This stage could begin with sharing your background and inner concerns — basically meeting the counsellor and building trust. Your joint efforts should concentrate on making any resistance conscious. Visualisations for relaxation and inner world contact and/or Gestalt exercises to integrate or 'own' symbols from the unconscious may be explored a little to support the development of trust. This also opens up the intrinsic interest in self-discovery which strengthens motivation for the healing work.

The second stage begins your self-exploration. You may move into some systematic relaxation and self-awareness on a physical level; possibly some dreamwork using simple ways to explore the main symbols in any recent or recurring dreams. Drawing on body outlines may be used to help locate and express pains or blocked feelings in the body.

Quite often you will be ready to burst with feelings and the session may move directly into the third stage involving emotional release processes. These could include bioenergetics, body focus methods and other emotional release processes that are designed to 'trigger' release of recent or past emotional pains. Some clients will want to move directly into a breathwork session.

Integration is the important fourth stage allowing time to rest and connect deeply to your awakened energy. This stage may include verbal sharing and assessing further support; journal writing, mandala drawing and relaxation.

During the fifth stage an emotional release counsellor may help you link your inner experience with new directions or new aims in your outer life. You should feel support for your creativity and expression of the new energy.

The final stage draws together all aspects of your work so far. You explore the link between personal healing work and journeying. As you gain trust, experience, interest and responsibility for your own healing, and as you have strong experiences of a freer, more alive energy state, you may begin to understand your inner healing work as a journey. While you may always have some specific personal healing goals, you will also begin to see that your healing and well-being has no limit.

◆

Reviewing personal growth after six months of ERC
A 45-year-old woman writes in her journal

My intention for my inner journey for these past months was to: 'Love and surrender to the life inside me — its ebb and flow and the changes it brings.' This intention intensified in its detail and became a wish to: 'be my own best friend, to comfort myself, to value and nurture my energy and support myself emotionally.' I did not anticipate that this wish would evoke the letting go of the external attachments of the Hurt Inner Child in order to focus within for nourishment and care.

To my surprise I found that to accept my own journey was a painful process. It meant that I could no longer let the hurt inner child manipulate others to get her needs met. The struggle was over. The task was now clear — to feel the pain of the hurt inner child and separate from it. The alternative was to go unconscious again, continue the 'hoo-ha' of distractions and not take responsibility for the quality of my relationships or my life. The more I allowed myself to have my journey I could allow others theirs. This was an unexpected gift of the healing.

I began to have a sense that I was waking up out of a deep sleep. Imagery of the court in Sleeping Beauty, asleep for one hundred years, was poignant in my consciousness. There was a sense of aspects of my life which had existed all along but I hadn't noticed them. It was as if the light was now switched on. Everywhere I looked in my life I could see how or where I had been asleep. The hurt inner child previously had total control of my life.

Transpersonal breathwork

Breathwork is one of the most dramatic and transformative emotional release processes. It is a powerful personal growth technique which uses strong breath as a way of connecting you to the depths of your inner world. The technique described here has been developed in Australia over the last fifteen years. It is based on the original Holotropic Breath-work™ of Dr Stan Grof and Christina Grof in the USA. 'Rebirthing' is a name for a similar process developed by Leonard Orr in the USA.

Breathwork is an emotional release experience that brings new energy or a 'rebirth of life'. It can be a therapy and a personal growth method that reconnects your unconscious memories and energies with your everyday waking consciousness. This gives great clarity and freshness to the way you live. Also, many of your attitudes and the problems you experience in life have a connection to your birth. Your birth was the first big struggle, the first separation. In a breathwork session your experiences can be relived, released and no longer influence you negatively. This leaves you free to face life in a new way.

Emotional release breathwork is described as 'transpersonal'. *Trans* means beyond or across. The extra energy that the breathwork awakens takes you beyond the personal, beyond the ordinary level of your consciousness. You may face personal problems then be able to contact a part of yourself that is beyond them. Breathwork raises you out of your normal, daily level so that you can see the pattern of your whole life. This non-ordinary state of consciousness allows your inner healer to work productively, unhindered by the usual defences and ego controls.

In a breathwork session you may access forgotten events from childhood. It is typical for someone to realise, 'Oh, that's why this is like it is now!' Past events now have a different meaning, or actually have meaning for the first time. Now you have some choice in your direction. New wishes emerge for future directions.

Breathwork opens up three realms of experience:
- Biographical — all the things that have happened to you and been felt since birth.
- Perinatal — relating to the time around your birth; within the womb, the birth itself, and the immediate post-natal experiences. This realm often links us into the transpersonal.
- Transpersonal — includes a very wide range of experiences, many not considered real in our culture. It involves expanding your awareness beyond your skin. You may

connect with the collective unconscious and many people experience a connection with the divine.

Breathwork sessions are usually conducted individually at first. When you gain confidence you may wish to join a workshop or work in a group. This provides even more energy and support.

I have found that breathwork sessions teach you who you really are under all your conditioning and social veneer. During a session you may deal with relationship difficulties, loneliness, anger and aggression, lack of meaning in life, sexuality, and much more. Some people remember and relive the power of love that they felt as infants. Most people remember things they have missed out on or sometimes violent events that surrounded them. It is the traumas you have experienced that play a big part in setting how you relate to others and your environment.

Through the breathwork you may experience the energy centres of your body powerfully awakening. Some people experience a flow of the lifeforce energy which they have never felt before. Sometimes your spiritual self speaks in images or symbols and gives powerful messages that bring new direction and healing.

One of the sad outcomes of carrying an overload of personal pain is that we cut off from our own sacred dimensions. And many people who work with the breath find that they come to their own personal deep reconnection with spirituality.

The breathwork technique itself is simple and natural. Unconsciously, to help yourself cut off from past hurts and to hold down unwelcome excitement, you reduced your breath. So in breathwork you open the breath again. It is an easy but dramatic reversal of the old constricted pattern. Relaxation and powerful music are also used to support surrender to the unconscious.

In a session you breathe fully, as deeply as possible, bringing your total energy to expanding the in-breath. The breath becomes deep, full, circular. This is called connected breathing. Your facilitator watches your breath very carefully and ensures you relax on the out-breath. He or she is encouraging you to go to your limits as you pull in the energy that is waiting in the air, ready for you.

You remain a witness to the internal events. Sensations, images, feelings, sights, sounds long buried, begin to surface. Sometimes emotions buried for years come right out in bursts of laughter or tears. You keep breathing and the tears transform. You move deeply through the personal experiences. Your facilitator may occasionally reflect back any feelings you share, but they will not interfere or explain or interpret. It is your time to 'stand under' your deep inner experience, in order to 'understand' in a totally new way. New meaning and explanations emerge, and your negative repeating patterns may become clear.

Your facilitator is there to support you in re-experiencing moments where you originally split off. They will assure you that complete feeling of any painful experience will be the healing of it. Their love and attention will help you face anything, express anything. There may be times when your fists will want to pound, your feet will want to kick. You will feel cushions ready. You enter the great pleasure of allowing yourself to explode.

Working this way, in a safe supportive space, with a fully qualified practitioner, enables you to reclaim who you were truly meant to be; it gives you the chance to remove the obstacles to living with our full potential. Transpersonal breathwork is described in more detail in my book *From Healing To Awakening* (1991).

◆

Self-criticism and breathwork
A 42-year-old man writes

It seems to me that nothing I do is good enough lately. I have been listening to this voice inside that is negative and critical. The night before my breathwork session I awoke at 3 a.m., with a clear knowing that my issue of not being good enough is connected to my father's attitude towards me. He never appreciated anything I did. Nothing I did ever got his recognition.

In my session I focussed on the increase I have felt in my self-criticism. Many tears came forth when I thought, 'Will it be all right?' — meaning will my work in the world turn out well, is my sense of purpose true? I could see that the childhood imprint that I am not good enough has smothered me — like a wet blanket. As I cried and released my anger towards my father, I felt the imprint, the negative issue, lift out of my body. Then I felt clean and clear and relaxed.

Differences between breathwork and rebirthing

There are numerous differences in what is currently presented around the world as rebirthing and breathwork. Although much good has come from the original forms of rebirthing there are several differences that should be made clear.

One major difference is the encouragement of catharsis in transpersonal breathwork sessions. Catharsis is a strong release of psychic, emotional and physical tension through sounds and movements. It is my belief that this is an important element in long-term healing work, and it is certainly supported in transpersonal breathwork sessions.

Some rebirthers from the Leonard Orr school are strongly linked to certain philosophical beliefs. A counsellor who tries to impose any beliefs on a client should be seriously questioned. Other rebirthers impose a rational cognitive viewpoint which implies that we can make choices about letting go of negative patterns. There may be a link here to the 'positive thinking' schools of thought. Our work with transpersonal breathwork shows that deeply embedded trauma affects energy flow, emotional flow, muscle tone and moods. Only a deep release of the long-held patterns can make a lasting difference, and result in new positive ways of living.

Rebirthing may also involve the questionable use of affirmations. These verbal efforts to correct old beliefs may indeed bring a positive feeling for the moments they are being used, but it is our experience that they do not bring deep lasting psychological change. Many clients, in fact, have been even more upset by feeling themselves a failure in living up to the affirmations given to them by a rebirther. There is a substantial difference in being given a phrase to repeat by someone else, and recognising from your own deep self-discovery a new truth that you would like to remember.

Some rebirthers imply that accessing traumatic unconscious memories from the past is not necessary but this is not a balanced view. Only fully feeling, remembering and expressing the past that has shaped you can bring long-term healing and integration of the unconscious and the conscious.

Transpersonal breathwork and the counselling that accompanies it are informed by the spiritual frameworks and psychological models expressed by Jung, Grof, Janov, Perls and many other pioneers of the personal growth movement.

From a professional point of view, one of the most serious differences between rebirthing and transpersonal breathwork is in the duration and depth of training considered adequate to qualify a practitioner. There are rebirthing training courses that could be considered extremely brief. Training in transpersonal breathwork, as part of the emotional release counselling studies, is a two-and-a-half to three-year course.

Those of you who wish to move on from the exercises outlined in this book and advance their self-discovery through breathwork would be advised to question the facilitator they intend to work with about training and background. Membership of the professional body (The Emotional Release Counsellors Association in each state) is a good indication of adequate training.

Individual breathwork sessions

Individual breathwork sessions offer a safe and confidential way to deal with personal problems. The trust that develops in one-to-one work brings a sense of safety, self-acceptance and the courage to face emotional pain.

Most of us have lived with alienation from our true self. In a breathwork session you have the time and space to be with yourself. For more intensive work individual retreat programmes are ideal. They give time for both intensive individual work and rest and integration — all geared to one's own needs.

In an individual programme the counsellor can call upon the methods most suited to support your present journey. This may include traditional counselling methods, Gestalt work, dreamwork, sandplay, transpersonal breathwork, emotional release processing and bioenergetics and de-armouring exercises.

In order to have time for sharing and integration, breathwork and ERC sessions need to be about two to three hours per private session. Clients are asked to bring a drawing book and crayons to explore mandala drawing as a way of expressing their inner experience. A personal journal is also useful for recording and integrating new observations.

Group breathwork

It is common to have your first breathwork experience privately with a qualified professional, but you can also begin with a group experience. The size of the group should be about ten to twenty people, working in pairs alternating in supporting each other. There should always be several highly experienced professionals supervising the sessions and assisting each participant to integrate their experience.

The mutual support of fellow seekers and the energy field created by the group greatly enhances the depth of the sessions. A workshop setting takes you away from the demands of daily life and gives space and time to focus within and share at length with newly found friends. Group workshops generally include some dynamic meditation work to activate your energy, bioenergetics work, and time to ask all the questions that bubble up for some time after a session.

◆

I am the creator of my life
A 46-year-old woman writes

I learnt that all this mental working out, travelling back over old ground, looking for how I (the hurt inner child) could have won, was very time consuming. This hurt inner child has kicked and screamed, resisted and struggled against the people, events and situations all through my life. Huge amounts of potentially creative energy have gone into futile workings out that took me nowhere. All these efforts to be conscious became useless as they exhausted and deadened me.

This insight was enormously liberating. This pattern of struggle, resistance and self-recrimination had dominated my life so far.

Gradually an attitude of surrender and acceptance came and I began to relax. I no longer was a child who had things happen to her.

I was able to accept that consciously or unconsciously I am the creator of my life and I began to agree not to look backwards with eyes of regret, clinging to the past. Messages and symbols came to remind me to 'be still and listen'.

Training in ERC

You may feel drawn towards becoming a facilitator of personal and spiritual healing. This evolves naturally when the results of your own quest meet the needs of those who have just entered their personal journey.

There are many links between the great current of present-day healing and the traditional methods of many so-called primitive cultures. Energy release, breathwork, bodywork, bioenergetics, emotional catharsis, surrender to the unconscious can all be found in Shamanic practice, North American Indian ritual, the all-night communal dances of the Kalahari Bushmen and in some Australian Aboriginal rituals and dance. We are rediscovering what has always been known!

Becoming a healing facilitator calls you to learn how to be emotionally open and energetically in flow. You need to be in a state of readiness, so that energy can work through you. Being a facilitator means experiencing grace, surrender and pleasure from coming back 'home', dropping your personal 'doing'. From this more open space intuition can operate; trans-personal energy, higher knowing — even love — can flow.

The role of therapist, co-journeyer, or support person brings many demands. You must know your own needs and fulfil them. Being deeply in tune with yourself ensures that nothing is projected on to clients or fellow seekers; you see them clearly.

Watch your ego constantly. Are you able to return to the seeker/self-healer within? Can you find again the humble, sincere part that keeps your own journey alive? Have you taken credit for growth in others and forgotten that you simply help them free their own natural healing forces?

Agreeing to be a healer means being stretched, coming close to the 'end of your tether' in giving to others. This demand extends your ability and stamina to give. It also calls up the extra energy you need in your search.

Healing requires some growing contact with your body and the energies that flow inside and around it. Becoming a healer demands a deeper and continual contact within. Living 'at home' means nourishing your body: dancing, resting, awakening the subtle energies, meditating, celebrating, making love. It may mean giving it special times with strong breath to release the past and quiet retreats to enter the now more fully.

To continue the journey towards becoming wholly oneself — as well as a helper — requires reminders. One final demand is that we frequently return to our own personal healing and continued growth. Most of us find that work with a regular group — with its deep sharing and the inspiration of seeing others grow — is the greatest support.

The number of such groups is growing. Together, we are creating a new sense of community, one based on supporting the natural movement towards wholeness.

Epilogue

Repair the past, prepare the future.

G. I. Gurdjieff from *Views From The Real World* (1973)

Future Directions

Some of the gifts I see this journey bringing are: clarity in self-perception and a clear view of the real situation around us; honesty with ourselves and with others; and, especially, the elusive quality called being.

At a certain stage of healing and after many self-discoveries, and many many experiences of centredness, you will achieve a growth in being.

Being is not a quality that is recognised by the world at large although this is slowly changing. Only those who have faced the challenge of being true to themselves, who have become to some degree undefended, and found some degree of stillness within, will recognise it. Being is not satisfying to your ego, but through it we can know the changes we need to make in outer life. And through being we change internally — right order is re-established in the psyche.

The Western world has regarded knowledge and external achievement as the main goals. The rate of growth of knowledge has outpaced, by a long way, the rate of growth of being, causing a serious imbalance within our civilisation.

The work of the healing journey redresses this imbalance in ourselves. This inner ability of presence, receptivity, clarity, seeing the truth — which we sum up as being — allows us to use knowledge in a wise and compassionate way. Our inner healing work helps us operate from a complete perspective or, in other words, body, mind and feeling working harmoniously. We are no longer content just to think our life; we want to be in it totally!

Although being is a great gift, it is an expensive one too. Every journeyer has felt how much inner healing work is required as payment. The changes that come from the experience and expansion of being may seem gradual, but they will certainly follow, bringing the essential nourishment we long for.

There are many exciting questions facing us, especially what to do with the new life this healing work releases. Some principles of the healing journey apply to the individual psyche, to ourselves, but how do they relate to the global situation?

Imagine the energy released in one strong ERC session, then multiply it by the millions of people on the planet! Repressed emotions use up a lot of energy! This energy, if freed, can be used in a creative way. Because people disallow their emotions they often become distant from a natural morality. This results in being distant from a feeling of what is right for the planet. There is widespread estrangement from spiritual realities and entrenched identification with a purely material approach to life.

Hatred and violence appear before us nightly on the television news. How often are these emotions the result of projected shadow qualities, the reaction to seeing in another our own fears, our own disowned negative parts? How much racial tension and violence results from these disowned and projected feelings?

When an individual or a community has lost touch with spiritual meaning, the whims of the ego dictate future directions. Whims of the ego usually revolve around self-protection and self-aggrandisement. For example, if I don't know that an exciting spiritual journey is possible — and waiting for me — I may choose a journey of wealth creation, or a journey of gathering political power, or I may simply wallow in the apparent meaninglessness of life. I certainly would not be fulfilling my personal and communal purpose.

The habitual repression of feelings and personal armouring in most modern cultures leads to an inability to find pleasure. Most of us fail to experience the pleasure of life. But since we need some pleasure to keep on living, we usually unconsciously attach pleasure to destructive, divisive ways of being and behaving. These negative ways are very hard to give up because they contain the pleasure of some release. Better law enforcement and bigger gaols, do not help. The question is how can chronically destructive people find authentic positive pleasure inside themselves and through that leave their old ways behind?

It starts with us. We must work free of the hurt inner child imprint that tells us we are helpless or powerless. We do not need a parental 'government' to supply all the answers.

Imagine the effect on the local community if all individuals were fully emotionally mature. Imagine the effect on our educational institutions and future society if all children were attended to on a deep emotional level and grew up satisfied? What if children grew up emotionally independent and able to give?

Imagine how society would benefit if the practice of educating and empowering parents-to-be included emotional growth practices and that the birth process became sacred. What a positive start it would be if every baby was welcomed into a conscious and caring, relaxed energy field.

What if every school had a counsellor with a beautiful, safe, private room for emotional release? What if distressed children received therapeutic guidance and healing support rather than punishment?

How would it affect our home life if parents had the opportunity to train in communication and active listening together with their children? What if children were encouraged to know their wonderful inner world? What if they were taught how to listen within for guidance and direction in their lives? What if they were regularly taught how to safely and effectively release pent-up feelings?

How would it transform our culture if business people were able to train in the skills of listening to their intuition and their conscience? What richness could be shared and reconciliation achieved if tribal people were able to learn new ways to reconnect to their own unconscious and their group unconscious to rediscover the basis of their authentic culture?

What if there were safe, beautiful, affordable places where those who felt lost, in emotional pain, could go for prolonged periods to allow their healing, with expert guidance?

In some way all of these dreams are happening now. All these 'what if's' are now becoming what is.

Further reading

Breathwork and Transpersonal Psychology:

Grof, Stanislav, *The Adventure of Self Discovery, Dimensions of Consciousness and New Perspectives in Psychotherapy and Inner Exploration*, State University of New York Press, USA, 1988

Grof, Stanislav, *The Holotropic Mind, The Three Levels of Human Consciousness and How They Shape Our Lives*, HarperSanFrancisco, USA, 1993

Pearson, Mark, *From Healing To Awakening: An Introduction to Transpersonal Breathwork*, Inner Work Partnership, NSW, 1991

Taylor, Kylea, *The Breathwork Experience: Exploration and Healing in Non-ordinary States of Consciousness*, Hanford Mead Publishers, USA, 1994

Overviews of the psyche and the healing journey:

Grof, Stanislav & Christina, *The Stormy Search For The Self*, J. P. Tarcher, USA, 1989

Johnson, Robert A., *The Psychology of Romantic Love*, Arkana, Britain, 1987

Jung, Carl Gustav, *Man And His Symbols*, Dell Paperback, USA, 1964

Jung, Carl Gustav, *Memories, Dreams and Reflections*, Fontana Paperback, London, 1983

Pierrakos, Eva, *The Pathwork of Self-Transformation*, Bantam, USA, 1990

Pierrakos, Eva & Thesenga, Donovan, *Fear No Evil: The Pathwork Method of Transforming the Lower Self*, Pathwork Press, USA, 1992

Personal development work:

Thesenga, Susan, *The Undefended Self: Living the Pathwork of Spiritual Wholeness*, 2nd ed., Pathwork Press, USA, 1994

Lowen, Alexander, *Bioenergetics: the revolutionary therapy that uses the language of the body to heal the problems of the mind*, Penguin Books, Britain, 1976

Perls, Fritz, *Gestalt Therapy Verbatim*, Real People Press, USA, 1969

Pierrakos, Eva & Saly, Judith, *Creating Union:The Pathwork of Relationship*, Pathwork Press, USA, 1993

Reich, Wilhelm, *The Function Of The Orgasm: Sex-Economic Problems of Biological Energy*, Simon & Schuster, USA, 1973

Childhood, birth and emotional development:

Leboyer, Frederick, *Birth Without Violence*, Alfred A. Knopf, New York, 1984

Janov, Arthur, *The New Primal Scream: Primal Therapy 20 Years On*, Abacus, Britain, 1990

Noble, Elizabeth, *Primal Connections: How our experience from conception to birth influences our emotions, behaviour, and health*, Simon and Schuster, USA, 1993

Pearson, Mark & Nolan, Patricia, *Emotional First-Aid for Children: Emotional Release Exercises and Inner-Life Skills*, Butterfly Books, NSW, 1991

Pearson, Mark & Nolan, Patricia, *Emotional Release For Children: Repairing the Past, Preparing the Future*, ACER, Melbourne, 1995

Reich, Wilhelm, *Children of the Future: On the Prevention of Sexual Pathology*, Farrar Straus Giroux, New York, 1984

Music that supports inner work

Here are a few suggestions for music that is very supportive of particular feelings and energies. Many selections are film soundtracks because film composers are usually required to focus on one emotion or one clear mood. Usually only certain tracks on the CD fit the mood category, so you will need to become familiar with the music before using it. (All music listed is available on CD unless specified as other.)

Tenderness:

Geoffrey Burgon, *Brideshead Revisited* television soundtrack
John Barry, *Somewhere In Time* and suite from *Indecent Proposal* soundtracks
Mark Knopfler, *Princess Bride* soundtrack
James Newton Howard, *The Prince of Tides* soundtrack
James Horner, *Braveheart* soundtrack (quiet tracks)

Grief, sadness, loss:

John Barry, *Out of Africa* and *Dances With Wolves* soundtracks and *Moviola* film theme compilation.

Anger:

Trevor Jones, *The Last of the Mohicans* soundtrack
John Barry, *The Black Hole* soundtrack available on record only.
Jerry Goldsmith, *Total Recall* soundtrack
Gustav Holst, *The Planets* suite (Mars)

Powerfully alive energy:

Vangelis, *Antarctica* and *1492* soundtracks and *Themes* film theme compilation
John Barry, *Dances With Wolves* soundtrack (stronger, louder tracks)
The Dervishes of Turkey (Sufi music)

Stillness, relaxation, letting go:

Ennio Morricone, *City of Joy* soundtrack (quieter tracks)
Terry Oldfield, *Cascade* and *Illuminations*
Brian Eno & Harold Budd, *Plateaux of Mirrors*
Patrick Bernhardt, *Atlantis Angelis*
Tony O'Connor, *Mariner* and *In Touch*
Alan Stivell, *Renaissance of the Celtic Harp*
Anugama, *Healing — Spiritual Environment*
Enya, *Memory of Trees*

Strong movement and celebration:

Sirocco, *Port of Call*, *Wetland Suite* and *Breath of Time*
Zorba The Greek soundtrack
Chris Spheeris, *Culture*
Mike Batt, *Caravans* soundtrack

Heroic:

Maurice Jarre, *Lawrence of Arabia* soundtrack
Vangelis, *1492* soundtrack (especially Track 2)
James Horner, *Willow* and *Legends of the Fall* soundtracks

Tribal rhythms:

Gabrielle Roth, *Totem*, *Ritual*, *Bones*, *Luna*, *Waves* and *Trance* (tapes and CDs distributed by: Spiral Booksellers, 269 Smith St, Fitzroy, Victoria 3065)
Prem Das, *Dreaming Drums*
Scott Fitzgerald, *Thunderdrums I* and *Thunderdrums II — All One Tribe*
Brent Lewis, *Earth Tribe Rhythms*

Where to find training and support

For contact numbers of qualified Emotional Release Counsellors and Transpersonal Breathwork Practitioners around
Australia or for information on personal growth centres,
workshops or training courses contact:

Mark Pearson
c/- Lothian Books
11 Munro Street
Port Melbourne Vic 3207

The Emotional Release Counsellors Association of NSW Inc.
c/- Patricia and Steve Nolan
The Inner Journey Centre
86 Toms Creek Road
Ellenborough NSW 2446
(065) 87 4356

The Queensland Emotional Release Counsellors Association,
Inc.
c/- The Portiuncula
173 Glenvale Road
Toowoomba Qld 4350
(076) 33 1383

Emotional Release Counsellors in Victoria
c/- Bernadette Wallis
PO Box 91
Caulfield South Vic 3162
(03) 9528 3014

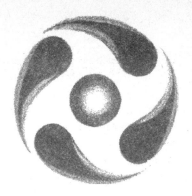

Glossary

armouring: permanent contraction of muscles into a fixed body stance (e.g. retracted pelvis, chronically expanded chest) see also de-armouring.

bioenergetics: specific exercises devised by Dr Alexander Lowen and Dr John Pierrakos which awaken and assist the flow of emotions and energy within the body.

centred: a state of focussed attention on the sensations in the body. Such a state enables you to become calm and more attentive.

chakras: potential energy centres which act as receptors and distributors for inflowing cosmic energy. There are seven chakra centres located along the midline of the body near the major nerve plexuses.

collective unconscious: a Jungian term which describes the existence of a common pool of memories available to all, no matter what race, spiritual tradition or era.

conditioning: a modification of behaviour learned through receiving positive and negative responses from people, society and culture. Usually conditioned behaviour replaces natural responses.

core: an area through the centre of the body, described by Wilhelm Reich, where energy circulates up and down. A very similar concept can be seen in Indian diagrams of the subtle body and energy channels.

de-armouring: release of chronic muscular tension which allows a flow of energy into those parts of the body that have been armoured.

defences: any method, technique or device that stops you feeling emotional pain. Defences can be organic — chemical, neurological, muscular and respiratory — or behavioural e.g. projecting, blaming, dumping.

ego: the educated part of the psyche that can organise and deal with the outer world. Your ego may have defences that are adopted and imitated in order to avoid emotional pain.

ego shift: occurs when the dominance of the ego is reduced and you are able to operate from a more essential part of yourself.

energy bodies: fields of energy that permeate and surround the physical body.

energy field: refers to human bio-energy which spreads beyond the skin and can permeate and deplete or stimulate another's energy.

eros: the energy of relating, sharing, mutual revelation and discovery.

hurt inner child: the part of the psyche that holds unhealed childhood hurts — sometimes described as a sub-personality. A complex of unfinished business from childhood, including incomplete emotions that were repressed, and emotional hurts such as feeling neglected or ignored. This complex operates through your life and creates a struggle to attain what was missing from childhood.

idealised self-image: an imagined ideal, learned in your early years, of how you should behave in order to gain acceptance and love.

individuation: a Jungian term for the psychological movement towards maturity and full self-realisation.

inner child: see hurt inner child.

integration: the organisation and assimilation of ideas, insights, memories and beliefs, in a way that leaves you feeling unified and complete.

interpretation: making sense of events and processes and ascribing specific significance to them.

karma yoga: a traditional way of spiritual practice through performing everyday activities while aiming for enhanced inner and outer awareness.

lifeforce: strong, alive, healthy bio-energy that is rarely fully utilised, yet holds the potential for full and vital life in the body, feelings and intellectual functions.

mandala: a drawing which is inspired by an emotional release experience or a period of being in contact with the unconscious. The drawing is expressed in a circle.

mirroring: reflecting and communicating a person's perceived emotional state to assist that person in connecting with their feelings.

perinatal: relating to the time around birth.

processing: involves expressing the hurts in a current problem in order to discover and experience this same hurt — or reactionary energy — which really belongs to a childhood event or trauma.

projection: the tendency to attribute to another person, or to the environment, what is actually within oneself.

rebirthing: a self-exploration process originated by Leonard Orr in the USA. The technique uses breathing and relaxation.

release: involves letting go some self-control so that a held-in feeling can be felt again, and transformed. Muscular contraction is relaxed at the same time.

repression: occurs when undesirable information is locked away from the conscious self.

resistance: not wanting to go forward with self-discovery or an inner healing process. Resistance can be conscious or unconscious. Resistance emerges as an attempt by the psyche to protect us from emotional pain.

shadow: a term used by Jung to describe any part of the human psyche that is suppressed and/or undeveloped. Shadow parts reside in the unconscious.

sounding, sounding out: the uncontrolled release of noises. This may include words and phrases, spoken or shouted, which have been held in the body for a long time.

transference: the transferring of childhood experiences, feelings or memories on to current situations.

transpersonal: *trans* means across, beyond. Transpersonal describes an inner world experience that opens a person beyond their personal issues; beyond their ordinary level of consciousness.

trauma: physical, emotional or spiritual wounding of serious magnitude. Traumas are frequently repressed and not integrated into your psyche.

trigger: someone or something outside you that stimulates your emotional reaction.

unconscious: the collection of memories, feelings, sensations and impulses that are stored in the brain and the body, that have an impact on behaviour, but of which you are not normally aware.

witness state: a calm emotional state of strong awareness, in which you can observe what is going on inside you.

Index of journal questions and exercises

Index